# RUN. TRAIN. RACE.

*Jim Fischer*

©2023 by Jim Fischer

All rights reserved. This book or any portion thereof may not be reproduced or used in any manner whatsoever without the express written permission of the publisher except for the use of brief quotations in a book review.

ISBN: 979-8-218-29472-4

Edited by Brittany Keller and Linda Reisor

Designed by Christine Fischer Studio, Wilmington, DE

Photography by Carlos Alejandro, Yorklyn, DE

Publishing assistance by The Happy Self-Publisher

Printed by Brilliant Graphics, Exton, PA

This book is not intended as a substitute for the medical advice of physicians. The reader should regularly consult a physician in matters relating to his/her health and fitness particularly with respect to any symptoms that may require diagnosis or medical attention.

The book is dedicated to my wife, Christine.
I would have never finished it without her love, time, and talent.

# RUN. TRAIN. RACE.

Practical distance running advice
for runners of all levels
based on 50 years of running,
teaching, and coaching

**JIM FISCHER**

With stories by friends and athletes
from around the world

# Contents

| INTRODUCTION | 9 |

# RUN

| THE FOUNDATION | 17 |
| GETTING STARTED | 17 |
| CLOTHING AND SHOES | 22 |
| RUNNING FORM | 28 |
| RUNNING RHYTHM | 34 |
| YOUR RUNNING | 36 |
| RUNNING SURFACES | 40 |
| LIFESTYLE | 44 |
| ENVIRONMENT | 50 |
| INJURIES | 56 |
| ILLNESSES | 63 |

# Contributors

CHRISTINE FISCHER

DR. ELISA M. BENZONI

SARAH HEINS

LIZ SWIERZBINSKI

BOBBY ZEIDLER

JOE COMPAGNI

ANDRE HOESCHEL

JANET AND ED DAVENPORT

STEVE PLASENCIA

LAINI MCGONIGLE

BILL LAFFERTY

# TRAIN

| | |
|---|---|
| **THE PREPARATION** | 69 |
| **TYPES OF WORKOUTS** | 78 |
| **SUPPLEMENTAL TRAINING** | 94 |
| **PUTTING IT ALL TOGETHER PERIODIZATION** | 107 |
| **TRAINING STRUCTURE** | 110 |
| **DOING WORKOUTS** | 118 |
| **USING YOUR WATCH** | 126 |
| **RECOVERY** | 131 |
| **MANAGING THE TRAINING CYCLE** | 137 |
| **LITTLE THINGS** | 139 |

# RACE

| | |
|---|---|
| **THE GOAL** | 149 |
| **PACING, PACING, PACING** | 151 |
| **RACING AS PART OF THE TRAINING CYCLE** | 153 |
| **BEFORE THE RACE** | 157 |
| **START** | 162 |
| **IN THE RACE** | 163 |
| **FINISH** | 171 |
| **RACING ON THE TRACK** | 176 |
| **RACING IN CROSS COUNTRY AND ROAD RACES** | 180 |
| **GETTING TO THE RACE** | 186 |
| **RACE DAY** | 190 |

---

**JIM BRAY**

**EMILY (GISPERT) WEAVER**

**ANDY WEAVER**

**MARNIE GIUNTA**

**ANNA PRYOR**

**NADINE MARKS DEMPSEY**

**NOEL RELYEA**

**MIKE DIGENNARO**

**BRITTANY KELLER**

**ART GULDEN**

**MELANIE AUBE**

**LAURA MCMILLAN**

**TRAVIS ADAMS**

**JIM BRAY**

**PATRICK CASTAGNO**

**VICKI HUBER-RUDAWSKY**

**ERIC ALBRIGHT**

**JOHN BRANNON**

**MARC WASHINGTON**

**ALLEN WAT**

**GARY WILSON**

**COLIN MCMILLAN**

---

| | |
|---|---|
| **KAREN (MANDRACHIA) PIACENTE** | |
| **REV. DR. NATE PHILLIPS** | |
| **DR. KATHRYN CARROLL** | |

| | |
|---|---|
| **WORKOUTS** | 195 |
| **ACKNOWLEDGMENTS** | 201 |
| **ABOUT THE AUTHOR** | 203 |

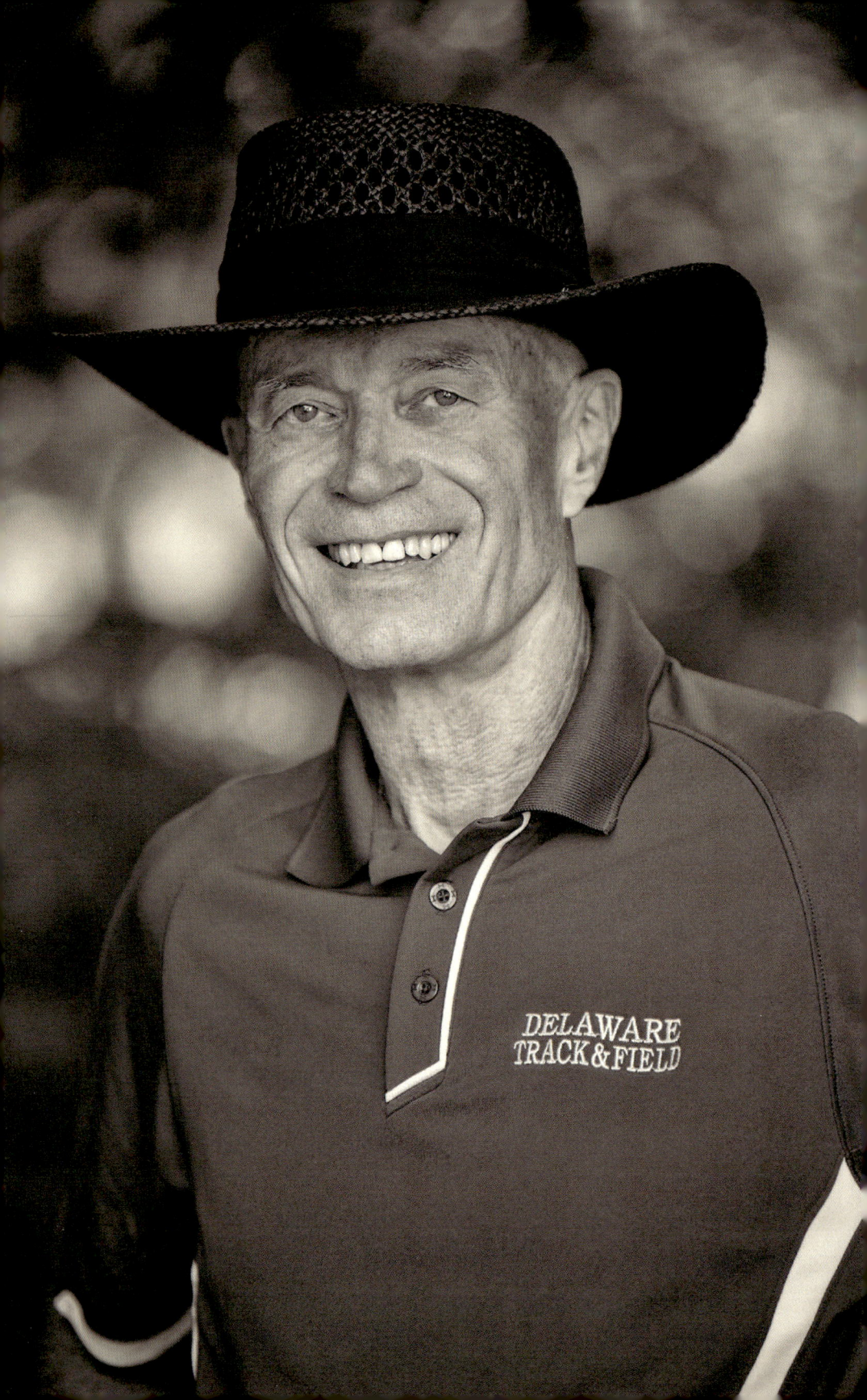

## INTRODUCTION

Distance running is such a simple activity, and that's what makes it so tricky competitively. There are no hidden ball tricks. There are no behind-the-back passes. There are no misdirected plays. It is all conditioning and flat-out work. It's sometimes said that our sport is other sports' punishment. But the results can be controllable, measurable, enjoyable, and satisfying. Running can be social, solitary, relaxing, exhaustive, casual, competitive, mind-clearing, thought-provoking, and exhilarating—whatever you want. At some point, almost every runner wants to enhance their running performance by striving to boost their fitness levels.

I began running on my high school's track & field team and competed as a collegiate athlete. I didn't run cross country until my senior year in college. I continued running road races for many years and continuously improved, learning as I went. With a sub 1:14 half marathon and a 2:43 marathon, I knew my running career would be limited. So, I shifted my focus toward working with others.

During my first year as a teacher, I replaced a track and field coach who had a heart attack one week into the spring season. That experience sparked a passion for the sport that grew stronger over time. I've had the pleasure of working with people at all levels of ability and fitness, and regardless of their starting point, the common themes have always been improvement and goal-setting. Through my work and studies, I've enhanced my running abilities, allowing me to increase my training and set more ambitious goals for myself. As both a runner and coach, I've learned a great deal from others, as well as through reading and trial and error.

I've been a teacher and coach, working with young and old. I thoroughly enjoyed teaching elementary physical education, junior high and senior high health, collegiate activity courses, safety, and measurement courses, as well as coaching all these age groups. I've worked with post-collegiate athletes as well.

I've coached cross country, track & field, cross country skiing, basketball, and football. I started a weekly workout session for adults and found that many people wanted to train but didn't know how to do it properly. Aside from weather issues and vacation weeks, I've enjoyed 40 years of these sessions ever since. The challenge of putting the training puzzles together for anyone, from beginners to elite athletes, has been intriguing and stimulating.

My goal for this book is based on an old proverb: Give you a fish, you will be fed today. Teach you to fish; you will be fed for the rest of your life. I could give you a workout that gives you something to do for today. Instead, I will give you fundamental principles of running, training, and racing, and you will understand what to do in the future. The information presented is my set of training rules. These guidelines, while important, lend themselves to situational and personal adaptations. As your fitness and performance improve, you will know what to do and what adaptations you can make to enjoy many successes.

Have fun!

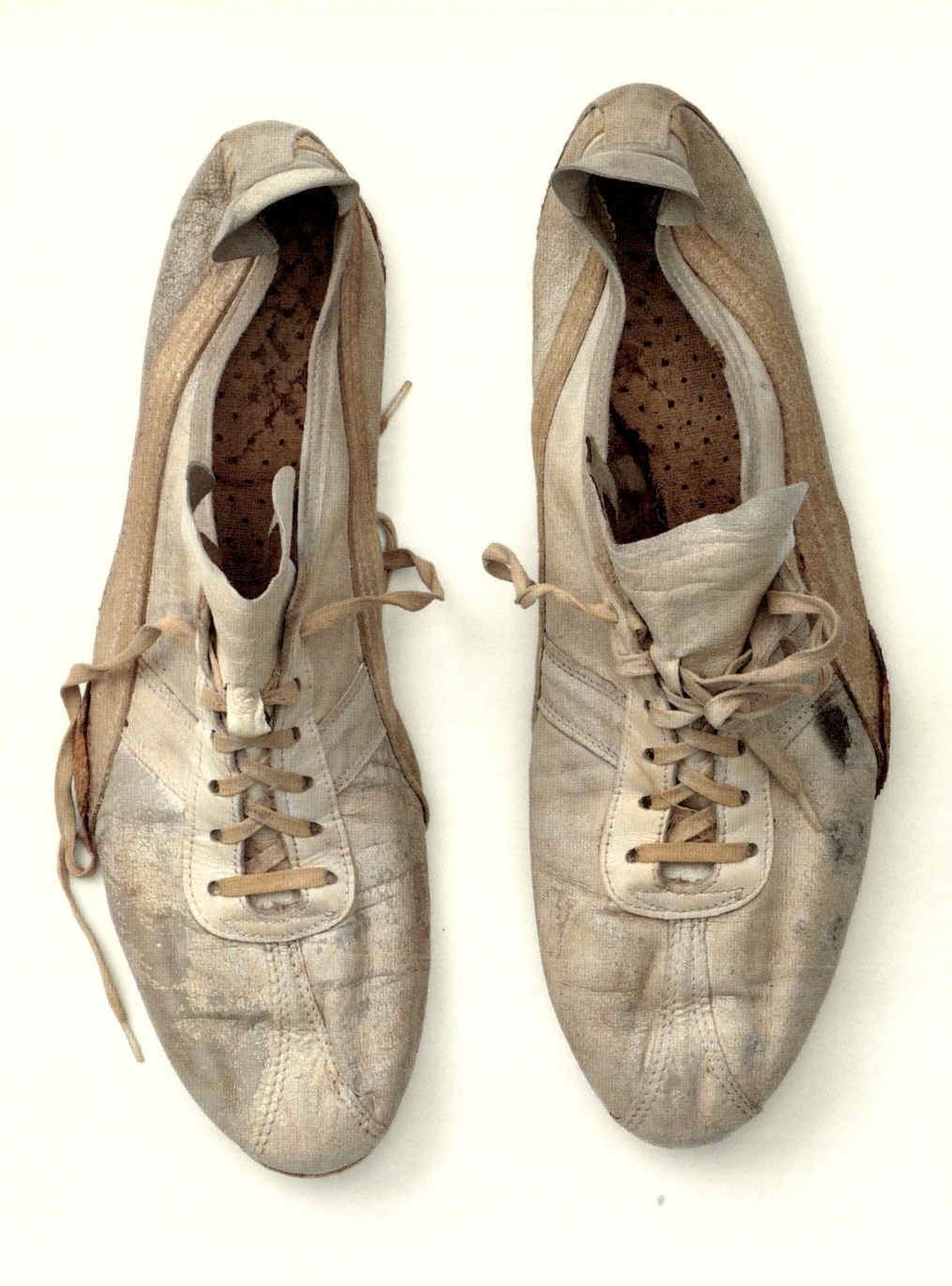

Jim Fischer
Running spikes worn at
Augsburg University
Minneapolis, Minnesota
1969–1970

## TRACK & FIELD STRETCHES

### Sitting/Lying

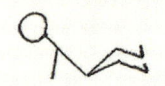

ABC's--drawing letters with the toes. The ankle joint is the only joint which is moved. This exercise is done to promote ankle flexibility.

Foot twists--forcibly rotating the ankle joint. Again, this is used for greater ankle flexibility.

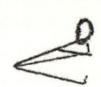

Straight leg stretch--can be done with legs spread, stretching toward one leg at a time, or with legs together. This stretches the back side of the legs and the lower back.

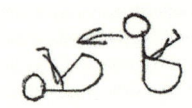

Roll-over--done in the egg or fetal position. It is used to help back flexibility.

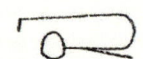

Back-over--legs straight to stretch, knees bent to relax while keeping the same general position. This stretches the lower back and hamstrings.

Single knee to chest--one leg held to the chest at a time. This exercise helps to stretch the lower back, buttocks, and the hamstrings.

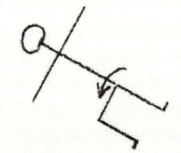

Side to side--one leg crosses over the other while shoulders remain flat. This is used for trunk and buttock flexibility.

### Standing

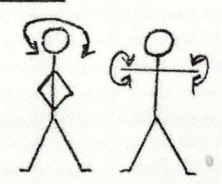

Rotations--rotating neck and shoulders. These are used to keep full range of motion.

# The Story of the Stories in this Book

**CHRISTINE FISCHER**

Several years ago, Jim and I were rummaging through some papers, and I found a Track & Field Stretches guide Jim had made in the 1970s. I fell in love with the simple icons that Jim illustrated to explain various stretching methods. They were quirky, not drawn with anatomical proportions, yet so expressive. I wanted to use these simple sketches in some way.

When I started to design Jim's book, I realized that his message isn't only great advice from an expert but also a conversation between a dedicated coach and an athlete. It isn't unlike the hundreds he's had with runners of all levels over his long career. He's maintained lifelong friendships with many of them.

I wanted to illustrate the incredible impact of these relationships on our life together. They have inspired runners to train, race, and become leaders in their professions, communities, and families.

We invited former athletes, coaching colleagues, friends, and family to share stories and artifacts that have inspired them throughout their running careers.

My dear friend Carlos Alejandro generously photographed the artifacts ranging from T-shirts and articles of clothing to treasured awards and stopwatches to 50-year-old racing spikes.

Some are composed in groupings around a theme; others are paired with a story highlighting a particular memory or experience. The stories are woven throughout the three sections of this book where they make the most sense. Jim and I are grateful to all the friends who have contributed to this project and hope the stories inspire our readers to recognize that running isn't just a sport; it's a lifestyle.

Jim Fischer's
Track & Field
Stretches guide
1970s

14  RUN. TRAIN. RACE.

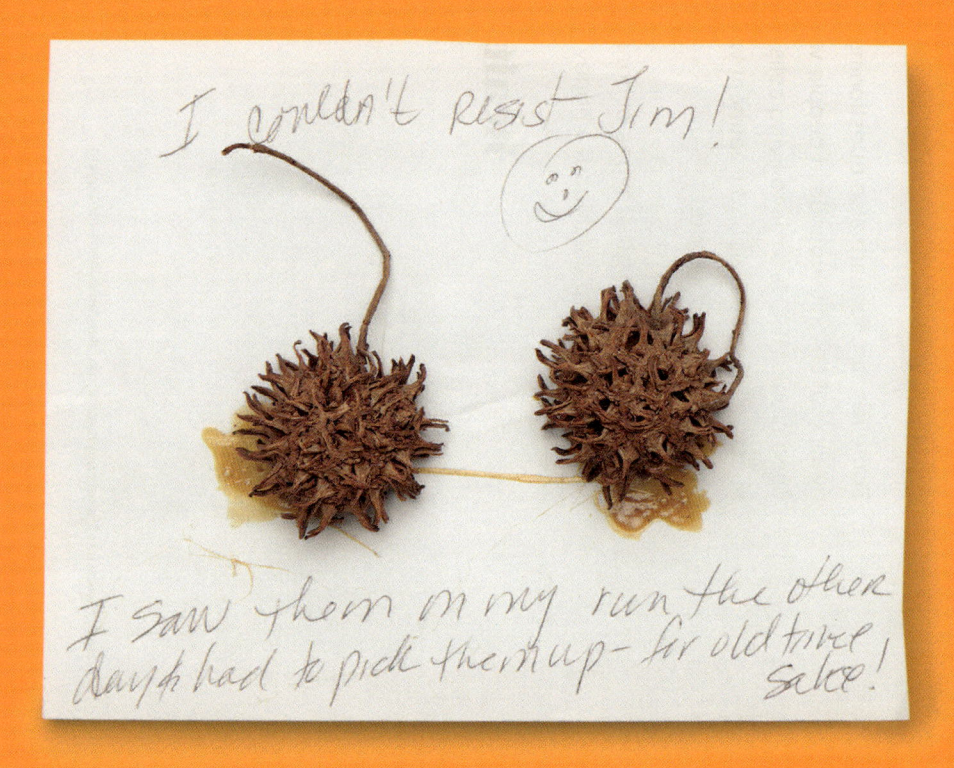

# RUN

I went to Boy Scout camp when I was young. One of the camp-wide events was a four-person relay—a runner gave the baton to a swimmer, who passed it on to two canoeists. I had some experience with running from my physical education classes and fitness tests, but I didn't expect that I would be anything special. The relay started, and we took off. I had the lead into the first hand-off by a good margin. It was thrilling, which led to me wanting to learn and practice more. It was the start of my journey. I discovered something I was good at doing, where I had a level of success and enjoyed myself. For over 50 years, running hasn't only been my career but a source of fitness, friendship, and fun. I ran countless workouts with friends I met at races and through the running clubs I joined. Many of my former athletes became professionals I admire. They are coaches, entrepreneurs, attorneys, engineers, medical professionals, and leaders. Through it all, I learned that running is more than a form of fitness. It's a positive force in overall wellness, self-esteem, and character.

**Dr. Elisa M. Benzoni**
**Sweetgum tree pods**
**Running partner**
**1994-1998**

**HERE ARE FIVE THINGS I WANT YOU TO REMEMBER AS YOU BEGIN YOUR JOURNEY IN YOUR RUNNING PROGRAM**

1. Get good shoes fitted at a running specialty shoe store and comfortable clothing appropriate for the changing seasons.

2. Run four days per week for 20-30 minutes. Run slowly and not very long.
Your progression should be slow.

3. Run with other people for company, enjoyment, motivation, and safety.

4. After a few months, pick a 5K to do with friends with the goal of finishing—slowly—and feeling good.

5. Be patient!

## THE FOUNDATION

Running is an activity that many of us have been doing since early in our lives. Running doesn't require much to participate. It is a great activity, simple to do, and provides a vehicle to reach cardiovascular health. Step out your front door, travel to the nearest State Park, or meet a friend in the next development and you can get in some exercise. Make this fun and enjoy the company, which will draw even more people to you and your group. People who have a good experience will tell others. First, check in with your doctor for a health physical like a high school or collegiate athlete is required to do. It is important that you know your limitations.

## GETTING STARTED

Be positive! Many times, people think about everything that could or has gone wrong. They become nervous about their current or future training or an upcoming race. Turn that nervous energy into excitement. It is a positive spin that can make one think about all that has gone well, giving a feeling of confidence. Picture yourself being successful.

Goals will help keep motivation elevated. The goals include consistency, weight loss, health, fun and socialization, improved performances, personal challenges, a mind-clearing oasis, planned destination races, fresh air, etc. Whatever your reasons, keep the targets moving. Find ways to keep things interesting and help provide direction for yourself.

In the beginning, your main goal is basic aerobic fitness. Your running can be measured in time or distance, whichever is comfortable, although time may be the easiest at first. Stay relaxed. The object is to move, and that's it. You can walk, run, or do a combination of both. More than likely, you will start too fast. So, tell yourself to go slowly. If you are worried about being able to sustain your run for any length of time, build in short walking breaks.

When I tell you to stay relaxed, I don't mean you should slow down. I want you to take a deep breath and drop your shoulders and arms. I want your upper body relaxed, with good form and rhythm. This will prompt your body to be fluid and in control.

Consistency is essential. For some, the hardest step is the first step out the door. Plan to run and then do it. Sometimes we add so much to the training program that it gets to the point that if there isn't enough time to get it all done, we skip the workout. Start with a manageable schedule and get comfortable with that. Add bit by bit to ensure the training doesn't get out of hand. If you have limited time, try to get something short done and return for a full workout the next day. Even a 20-minute easy shake-out will be better than nothing. It will help reinforce the habit.

The basic goal for people starting out should be a minimum of 20 to 30 minutes of activity on four days each week. Some use a schedule of Monday-Wednesday-Friday-Saturday or Tuesday-Thursday-Saturday-Sunday or other schedules depending on their life. Whatever you do, make it a schedule you can live with most of the time. This will give you the basic amount of exercise to improve your cardiovascular system.

I'll assume you want to run, at least part of the time. If running all the time is difficult, start by walking and running in a ratio. You can use time as your guide or use something as simple as telephone poles or streetlights. Start with as little as running to one pole and walking through the next three. Repeat this as the weeks go on until you are comfortable progressing to running two poles and walking two poles, then three poles running and one pole walking, and so on. Don't go too fast or too long. Take a walking break to refresh before you get so fatigued that you must walk. Get comfortable and increase at your own rate. You can use time or distance to measure your training. Finish feeling like you could have done more rather than feeling like you should have done less. Don't struggle. Keep your breathing natural and relaxed, never forced or strained.

Change your running routes often. The variety will be invigorating. You can explore. It is also essential for safety reasons so someone with nefarious purposes won't identify your pattern and schedule. Ensure your new route is safe regarding traffic, animal concerns, and personal safety. There are a few other things to remember. Try to train with another person. Listening to music makes running enjoyable but may limit advanced warning of any danger. Run in well-lit areas at night wearing reflective material and stay clear of overgrown paths. Carry an I.D. with medical info. Carry a phone. Limit your jewelry. Tell someone where you are going. Run against traffic. Carry a noisemaker and report harassment. There are other things you can do to protect yourself. This list is a good start.

Keep a log or journal. You can check progress from week to week, month to month, year to year. Reviewing the workouts and training patterns can indicate what does and doesn't work for you. There may be indicators to show what led to an injury or illness. There may be memories of great training periods and races that you will want to reference or remember. One useful tool is a wrist stopwatch, a watch with a GPS, or an app so you can monitor the workouts.

Plan to run a race. The goal for the first race is to finish—and that is it! Being around the race site will familiarize you with the registration lines, bathroom issues, chips, the start and finish areas, drink stations, etc. Your performance goals will come later. In the beginning, it is about finishing, feeling good, and being proud of your accomplishment!

Sarah Heins
Running log
2019-2020

# Running Recorded

**SARAH HEINS**

Every morning, I awake before sunrise and within a few minutes of crawling out of bed, I am racing down empty streets—my heart beating loudly and my feet pounding on the hard ground. Some days I run freely, allowing myself to travel at the pace my legs set for me, while other days, I complete regimented speed intervals, playful fartleks, or rhythmic tempo runs. Each and every one of these workouts is logged in my tattered training log, a simple spiral notebook that records the running rhythms that shape the course of my day and the structure of my week. These logs are written with intricate detail—meticulously outlining the mileage and paces of every training session, cataloging the exercises I complete during my post-run strength workouts, and describing my thoughts and experiences on each day's session. Furthermore, my training logs keep track of the mileage on my running shoes, the weekly and monthly totals of my training miles, and my personal-records in time-trials and races.

More than tracking my running metrics, my training logs also serve as an intimate history of my progress as a runner, holding the story of my growth, improvement, and evolution as an athlete. Through these logs, I can see where I first added weekly long runs to my schedule, remember when I ran my first interval workout on a track, and take note of just how many tempo-runs I have completed over the years. Like a diary that contains someone's deepest thoughts and emotions, these training logs hold on to a core part of who I am, containing within their pages the story of my life as I run through each and every day.

**RUN. TRAIN. RACE.**

## CLOTHING AND SHOES

Clothing and shoes should be next on the list. Your choice of clothes can reflect your style. There are some important considerations. On hot, sunny days, wear lightweight and lightly colored clothing. Clothing that absorbs sweat, such as cotton, can become heavy and uncomfortable and cause overheating. Instead, opt for dry-fit or moisture-wicking clothing that propels sweat away from the skin. On cold winter days, sweat-wicking clothing can be just as important. Wearing layers of clothes for wicking to keep the skin dry and warm with an outer wind block layer is essential. Wearing layers lets you take off or put on items to regulate your comfort. Also, be aware of clothing needs during the changing seasons, such as from winter to spring. With the weather changing frequently, I prefer taking too much. If you don't have it, you can't wear it.

Pay attention to the socks you wear. Many wick moisture away, and some prevent blisters. Old school socks can be cheap and easy to find, but they can lead to future blister trouble. Some socks are thin, and some are thick. Wear what feels most comfortable. Be aware that the thickness of your socks may impact your shoe size.

Buy good shoes. Shop at a store where the knowledgeable staff will help you select the right shoes for you. Try them on at the end of the day when your feet are most swollen. If shoes are too tight, circulation could be impaired, and there could be nerve damage. If they are too loose, support may not be in the correct place, or there could be a lack of stability, especially lateral stability. Don't buy your shoes too short. Try to have up to a half inch of space at the end of the shoe. They should be comfortable enough to prevent an injury or for you to lose concentration thinking about ill-fitting shoes. You want support, cushioning in the front and back of the shoe, the correct length and width, shape, a strong heel cup and counter, a flexible sole, a wide toe box, breathable material, the proper shape and position of the arch, and the right shoe for the type of running or racing you will be doing.

Some shoes are sturdy and grip well for trails, regular training shoes for doing the bulk of your mileage, light training and racing shoes for workouts and competitions, spikes for track and cross country races, and cross-training shoes for doing supplementary work in the gym. Running shoes are purposely more flexible than basketball or tennis shoes to limit stress on the Achilles tendon and calf muscles while being stiff enough to maintain support. The perfect color may be one of your desired qualities, but it is far down on the priority list. People with high arches, who are heavier, or who land heavily would generally need a more cushioned shoe. People with flat arches or who roll toward the inside of their foot (pronate) need a shoe with solid arch support that emphasizes motion control. Wide shoes on narrow feet will be sloppy and narrow shoes on wide feet will be restrictive and cramped. Walk and jog around the store in the shoes to check fit. After you buy a pair, walk around in them for a couple of days to help break them in, giving the shoes time to conform to your feet before using them in a workout or race.

Buy new shoes on a regular basis. Shoes typically last from 250 to 500 miles before they start to deteriorate. Log the total miles on them to know when it is time to change. You may have to change them sooner if you also wear them as casual everyday shoes. They may look great but not give you the support and cushioning you need. One indication that a change of shoes might be necessary is the onset of minor injuries. Generally, keep shoes for no more than six months, preferably three to four months, regardless of mileage. People who run 100+ miles per week need to change often.

Having two pairs of shoes and alternating them is a good idea. Shoes can take up to 48 hours to completely dry out. If they get soaked, stuff them with paper to help dry them inside and out. You can wash them, but don't dry them in a dryer. Most people find a type of shoe that they like and buy that shoe over and over. One idea is to have one pair new and another slightly worn to avoid consecutive workouts on worn shoes.

The alternative idea is to buy two different brands of shoes, both of which fit and are comfortable. They may put different stresses on the feet and legs, giving a slightly different feel and working out other parts of the leg muscles.

Many have taken to barefoot and minimalistic running, the theory being that the foot and the stride pattern are more natural. It isn't for everyone, although many have found success where they had previously struggled. For many years, I've recommended that barefoot running be used in small doses as a training tool to strengthen the muscles in the feet and lower legs. The downsides are overworking the muscles and exposing the feet to whatever is on the running surface. This is an individual decision. Consider the options to find what is best for you.

Spikes, racing flats, and lightweight training shoes give people that "fast" feeling when running a race or doing an intense workout. They are lighter than the typical training shoes and are generally worn tighter than training shoes. These may break down quickly, and their wear should be monitored closely. Make sure they provide you with the support and cushioning you need. Many also have a lower heel height. This can cause the calves to become tight and stiff as rocks. Early in the season, wear the low-healed shoes for a small part of the workout and gradually increase their use. Maintaining flexibility and progressively getting used to the low heels will help. Wear them in practices early and often.

One last thing to consider is how many people tie their shoelaces, crossing the laces next to the sock/foot. If you have an irritation on the top of your foot, it would be best to go down the eye hole and cross the tongue on the top of the side panels so the laces don't directly touch the sock or shoe tongue.

Your feet are the foundation for running. Investing in the proper running shoe is important in protecting your body from the impact of running.

Liz Swierzbinski
Store Manager, Delaware Running Company
UD Athlete 2005–2009

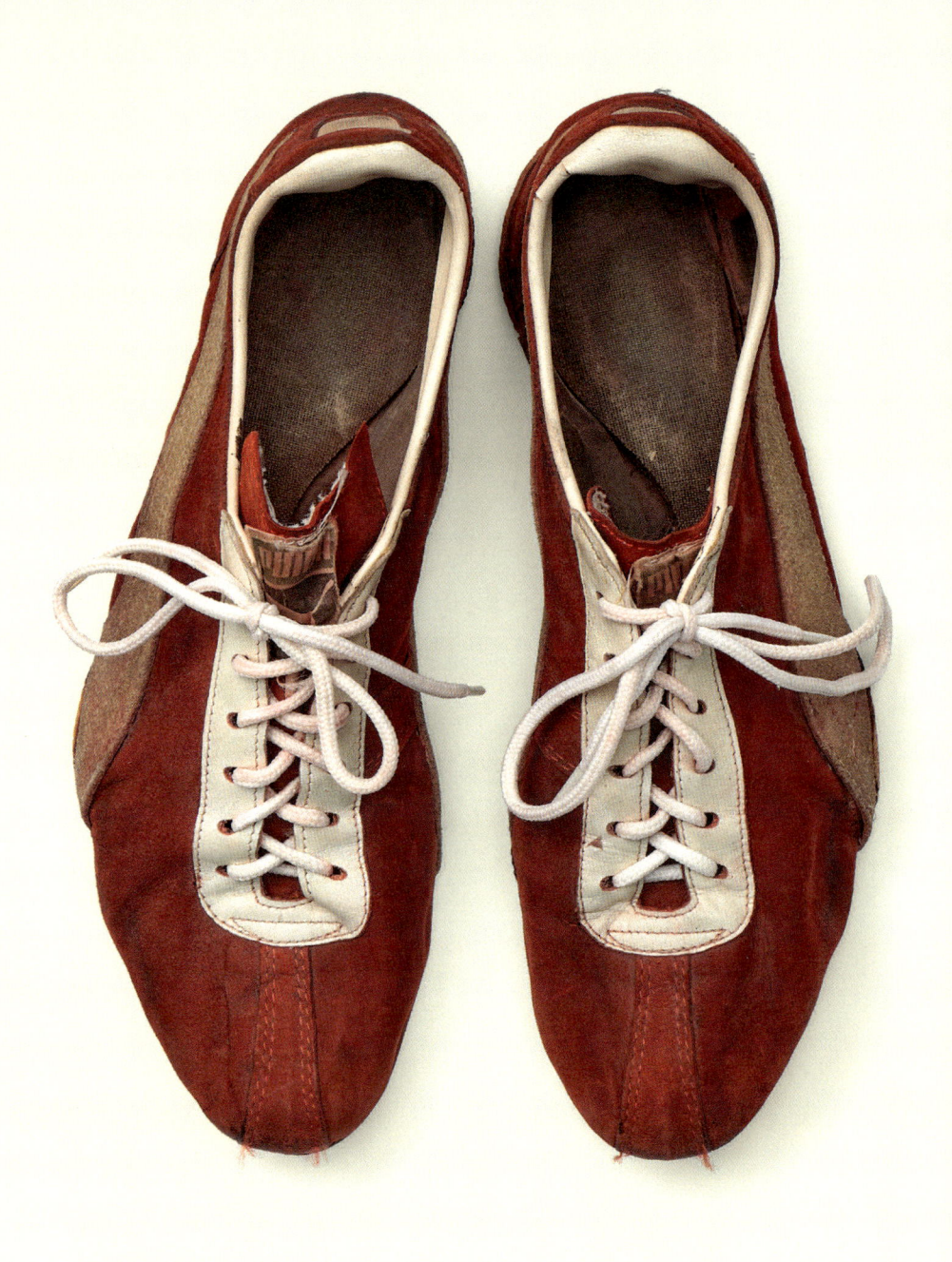

Bobby Zeidler
Cooper HS athlete
Running spikes
1975

# My First Pair of Spikes

**BOBBY ZEIDLER**

For much of my sophomore year in high school, I recall using lots of white athletic tape to salvage a pair of badly torn and nearly unusable track spikes that someone was throwing away.

The next year, I progressed by borrowing spikes for track meets from other teammates. The following year, it was 1975, and it took 20 hours of washing dishes at $1.62 an hour to purchase these spikes.

I recall the thrill of wearing, running, and racing in these spikes on a synthetic track. That may sound simplistic, but most of our races and practices were on cinder tracks. When these spikes were worn, it gave the feeling of being faster; it was like running barefoot. Depending on the track surface, we needed to have various lengths of spikes. If we had the improper spike length, we could risk disqualification or ruining the track surface. So, along with these expensive new shoes, I needed to purchase more spikes. I was no longer washing dishes at the Pancake House, so I was dependent on the distance runners community spike box. This is where we hunted for the best repurposed and sharpest metal spikes ranging in sizes from 1/8" up to what looked like 3" nails. Operating like a surgeon, we installed them with a small crescent wrench.

Years later, as a Dad, I was given the gift of seeing our son wear my old spikes. Giving them to wear for the first time at his middle school track meet in 2008; all of his teammates thought that these retro spikes were so awesome.

These spikes hold the memories of and represent a season of my life spent with my best friends and the best coach I ever had in Coach Fischer. Nowadays, these spikes hang on a hook in our basement. They are a reminder to me of a book I have read that speaks of living life in a way that we are to run in readiness and throw off anything that hinders us from running the race set before us.

## RUNNING FORM

There are basic form techniques and details that you want to remember. Feel light when you run, not heavy trudging. You shouldn't struggle at all while running. This is about rhythm, relaxation, balance, coordination, flexibility, and posture. Bad form and poor rhythm mean you will work harder than others to get the job done. Start slowly and control the length and intensity of your run. Stay "tall" as you run. I don't mean that you should be upright stiff. Just be erect and hold a good posture. This will make you more efficient, help your breathing, and limit things that will hurt your performance. Your form will become more challenging to maintain the farther you run and the more fatigue sets in. You can't think about your form every minute. Occasionally, check in with your form to assess how you are doing during your run.

For runners, breathing is a good thing. It's the way we get oxygen so we can function. People have recommended a variety of rhythms to use to be more effective and efficient. My main emphasis is that breathing should be relaxed. During a run, you may get to a point where your breathing is labored, and you start to struggle. To get back to a controlled, relaxed rhythm, you may need to slow down, relax the chest muscles, drop your shoulders and arms, and relax your mind.

Your chin should be level or slightly down, not tipped back, and your face and neck muscles should be loose. Grinding your teeth is a no-no. Tension in the face and neck usually leads to tightening of the whole upper body. Your chest should have little movement, not stiff, but not rotating. Arms should swing from the shoulders, and generally, the hands shouldn't cross the body's center line on each swing with the elbows swinging close to the body. Some runners hold their hands closely against their chest. That can be efficient. However, if the arm movement is too restricted and rigid, it can affect the normal running rhythm and breathing. The shoulders are down, and there is minimal trunk rotation. Hunching your shoulders wastes energy.

Take a breath, drop your arms and shoulders, relax briefly, and return to your normal form.

You don't want your arms driving back and forth, looking like a choo-choo train. The arms are held at approximately ninety degrees but not stiff. The angle at the elbow is slightly less than ninety degrees in front of you and slightly more in the back. The harder and faster you run, the larger the arm swing. In a sprint, the hands might get as high as the nose in front, and the elbows might get close to shoulder level in the back. Hands and fingers should be loose and lightly cupped, not tight in a fist or floppy. I've used a string wrapped around the two hands to keep them from flying everywhere and a rolled-up piece of paper to remind runners not to tighten their hands. Tight jaw, neck, and hands lead to tight arms and shoulders, which lead to restricted breathing and movement. Again, if someone tells you to relax, that doesn't mean slow down. It means relaxing the muscles in your face, neck, shoulders, arms, hands, chest, and back. Maintain good posture. Get back into a good rhythm. Save energy.

Run tall! You want your legs, knees, and feet preferably all going in the same direction—forward and straight. The pelvis is in a neutral position. Your body should have a slight forward lean, not by bending at the waist, but a lean that starts from the ankles. Too many times, runners bend at the waist or "sit" with their butt back as they run or hollow their back because it is easier. It isn't efficient! These will shorten your stride, making you biomechanically inefficient and possibly restricting your breathing. Muscle weaknesses and imbalances, bad coordination, wide hips, and body misalignments cause deviations from running straight. Some you can and should fix. Body structural issues may cause other problems and those you can't and shouldn't fix.

Another thing to look for is the position of the knees each time you are in single-leg support, and they cross next to each other. If the knees are at about the same level, that's great. It means your hip strength is good.

But, if the knee of the free leg, the one not on the ground, is much lower than the other knee when they cross, that's a problem. The knees and the hips should be level. The hips should also be square in the direction of travel. Under the watchful eye of a knowledgeable coach or having a gait analysis, some of these problems can be corrected.

There are many discussions about where the foot should first contact the ground. The point of contact depends on walking or running, speed, body structure, etc. You don't want hard heel contact, slapping, and pounding. If you make loud sounds every time one of your feet hits the ground, you aren't moving efficiently. Walking can produce forces from one to three times your body weight into the ground while running can create forces from two to eight, sometimes even ten times your body weight, depending on your efficiency.

Running is an explosion with each step. You want to spend as little time on the ground as possible. The push needs to be forward and not pop up in the air. You need to have more control over ground contact. While first contact of the foot can be anywhere from the heel to toe, usually, the foot rolls from the outside to the inside. Think of the foot as a ball rolling and not a board hitting flat. A flat, hard foot strike with a strong impact can cause excessive upper body rotation, injuries by the impact of those forces, and a lot of time spent on the ground. Strengthen your legs and shorten your stride. Try to get your foot strike under your center of gravity so you aren't working against yourself.

Many things will cause you to lose control of proper body mechanics: fatigue, compensation for the lack of strength, poor conditioning, hard training, overworked muscles, and lack of recovery. We all need to be vigilant. Having someone you trust watching you helps you adjust and maintain good form.

Many people, especially beginners, lock their shoulder joints, and the rotation of their upper body creates the illusion of an arm swing. They rotate their upper body around a vertical axis. This occurs due to incorrect form, lack of strength, or trying too hard. Relax and unlock the shoulder joint, letting the arm swing from the shoulder, not the rotation around the body's vertical axis. The chest shouldn't be stiff but can move slightly back and forth. Remember, run with good form—run tall, keep your upper body relaxed, and swing your arms from your shoulders. Run at an easy and comfortable pace. Stay relaxed and don't struggle. Keep your breathing and upper body open.

Just because a person looks like they have an awkward arm swing or upper body rotation doesn't mean it always should be or can be fixed. Movements and actions in the lower body because of structure, like a leg length discrepancy, a genetic restriction, or a limitation of some sort, can cause a reaction in the upper body, which is compensation needed to balance what is happening in the lower body. This may be a compensation that needs to happen. Tightness in the upper body can restrict the fluidity in the lower body. Working on little things to make you more efficient might lead to discovering whether other larger things can be tweaked.

Keep your foot plant under your belly button, your center of gravity. It is like running down a line with each foot landing on it. The foot plant doesn't always end up directly beneath the belly button when people walk. As you get faster and start to run, the pattern of steps develops into a single line.

Some people shift their weight from one foot to the other, bobbing their way from side to side. As part of this, the center of gravity (belly button) shouldn't move from side to side in a zig-zag movement. This should be corrected. The belly button must go in a straight line.

# A Career in Coaching

**JOE COMPAGNI**

My below-average times in high school meant that I received exactly zero recruiting calls. Wait—that's not true. I did receive one. It was from Coach Fischer. He surely only called, though, because I called him first, asking about the team. After hearing of my short and unimpressive high school running efforts, his message was simple: if I wanted to give it a shot, I could join the cross country and track & field team at the University of Delaware. That was all I needed to hear. I was in.

Four—well closer to five—years later, I had made some small contributions to the team, had the honor of being a captain for cross country, made lifelong friends, and developed a deep appreciation for our sport through the opportunity he provided. My story isn't that unique, and one that's shared in many ways by hundreds of student-athletes who were part of the program in Coach Fischer's 30 years of leading the program. He did so with a combination of grace, integrity, toughness, diligence, and humility that's unmatched.

Coach Fischer's impact in the state of Delaware and well beyond is immense. How many of his student-athletes went on to coach and are still coaching now? How many benefited from his fair-handed and knowledgeable advice and lead a better life thanks to his guidance? How many others were students in the courses he taught and gleaned some wisdom that they continue to share every day?

His Minnesota roots might lead Coach Fischer to tell you that what he has done was no big deal. Those of us fortunate enough to have spent some time with him know that it is, in fact, a very big deal.

Joe Compagni
**Monmouth University Coach**
UD athlete 1983-1987
**Monmouth University
Cross Country Invitational
T-shirt, 2016**

# 22ND A[NNUAL]
# MON[MOUTH]
# UNIVE[RSITY]
## CROSS COUNTRY

**2016 - HOLM[DEL]**

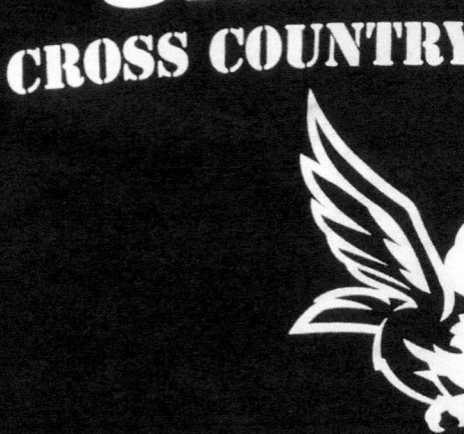

NNUAL
# MOUTH
# RSITY
Y INVITATIONAL

DEL PARK

## RUNNING RHYTHM

It is common for people to want to know the pace of their running. You must learn pace so that you can plan. Additionally, you should eventually learn to feel pace without the aid of a watch. You will hear people tell others to listen to their bodies. This is important. But you must know and understand what you are listening to hear. Awareness comes through experience. Pay attention.

Your effort on any particular day will determine how fast or far you go. But technically, when computing running speed or velocity, two things determine how fast you will run: stride length (distance traveled with each step) and stride frequency (number of strides taken per minute). A higher stride frequency usually means a decrease in stride length, at least at first. Running is, for the most part, a pushing activity. It is inefficient, energy-sapping, and extremely fatiguing to reach out in front of yourself, landing well in front of your body's center of gravity, thus pulling your body forward.

Training will help strengthen you so that your "push or explosion" on each step will be stronger and more dynamic, making each stride longer. The push should have a much larger horizontal component than a vertical one. At the same time, through practice, you can work to increase the number of strides taken each minute, improve your running economy, and reduce the ground impact forces, hopefully lowering the incidence of injuries. We all have limits to what our nervous system will do for us. Just work to maximize what you have.

You may need to shorten your stride to make this happen. The stride length will increase as you become more comfortable with an increased rhythm. In a study of elite marathon runners, as they fatigued during the race, the athletes showed a decreased stride length with little change in stride frequency.

Jack Daniels, an internationally recognized coach, in his book *Daniels' Running Formula*, noted that he studied elite runners and found that the stride frequency most identified among high-level athletes is generally around 180 steps per minute. This study was limited to elite runners. Not everyone in the world will have the same stride count, and inexperienced athletes will probably have trouble getting to that number. This optimum number will vary from person to person depending on experience, the speed and intensity of the run, form, body type, and so on.

A shorter, quicker stride frequency can help limit injury-causing overstriding and high impact forces. Long-term, faster turnover can lead to better speed as you get stronger. Rather than counting every step, counting the number of times your left foot hits the ground in a minute and multiplying by two is easier. You may be far from the stride frequency of elite runners, but it would be good to practice increasing yours regularly. Poor running mechanics, lack of dynamic strength, or fatigue can cause you to spend too much time on the ground. You want to propel yourself forward and forcefully get off the ground quickly.

While practicing a quicker stride rhythm, you might also address a good leg action. On the front side of the stride are knee lift and foot plant. On the back side of the stride are push-off and knee bend. For many, after the foot leaves the ground behind their body, the leg and foot just kind of dangle there for a fraction of a second before moving forward to take the next step. Practicing a quicker rhythm may help alleviate that hesitation, making the movement more efficient. Strive to bend your knees at the back of your stride. A straight leg is a long pendulum, slower, while a bent leg is a short pendulum, faster, with a larger arc of the leg swing.

## YOUR RUNNING

Your daily workout should include a short warmup jog, dynamic range of motion exercises, light stretching, another short jog, and striders on the days of intensity workouts, and then start your reps or run. Following the main part of the workout, do a warm-down jog, relaxed striders, strength and core work, and stretching.

Getting warmed up is an essential part of running to prepare the body for the upcoming activity. The circulatory system prepares to deliver fuel and oxygen to the cells, and muscles become more pliable. The warmup in the winter may have to be longer than in the summer and be continuous with very few rest periods when the muscles can quickly become cold again. Warmer weather may give you more flexibility. But you'll notice that as you work harder and harder, especially in hot and humid weather, the body's core temperature will rise higher and higher. If the core temperature gets too high, performance may suffer. This may also be a safety issue.

One day each week, try to run a little farther. If you are still determining if you can go farther, split your run into two runs or take water or walking breaks to get refreshed.

As the weeks go on, gradually progress the volume and intensity of your workouts. During a training run, take a walking break before you are so tired that you must walk. Don't struggle. Progression in your training should be gradual. You will work on slowly increasing the length of time that you run and the intensity at which you do it. This process is measured in months and years, not days and weeks. The long-term, general progression that I would use to increase your fitness is first to increase the number of days you run, second to increase the length or duration of the run, and lastly, increase the speed or intensity. Don't get caught up with increasing anything too quickly. Start with easy, controlled running, building up over time, letting muscles, tendons, ligaments, bones, and joints get used to the activity and keep

The old adage "if some is good, more is better" doesn't always hold with training. Be patient.

progressions slow. This is a process. Don't rush it. Adding duration and intensity at the same time can lead to problems. Also, the adage "if some is good, more is better" doesn't always hold with training. Be patient.

Don't try to make up for lost or missed days of training. Here is where your consistency will pay off. A few days off won't hurt if you have been running regularly. You may feel sluggish for the first few days until your fitness and rhythm return. Don't force your training. That good feeling and rhythm will come back.

Working hard is where everyone puts their emphasis. Unless the body has time to rebuild itself back to where it was and stronger, all the training will lead to a downward spiral. Some people will take longer than others to recover from the same workout. Ask yourself, does a run make you feel better or worse? Right away, you may say worse. Looking back a day or two or a week or a month, do you feel stronger or weaker? This is another scenario in which listening to your body is essential.

If you have heavy legs or want to recover after any workout or race, give yourself time, light running and activities, lie on your back with your legs propped up, eat a colorful plate including carbohydrates, fats and protein, hydrate, cross-train, stretch, swim, walk, massage, rollers, soak in a cold whirlpool, ice massage, contrast showers, use compression sleeves, mental relaxation exercises, use a slant board, put your feet up on a pillow, and rehydrate to get yourself back to feeling better. Even electro-stimulation and ultrasound can be used. Check your morning pulse rate to see if it is elevated from where it usually is. If it takes longer than 24–48 hours to recover, you may have had a tough workout or gone too long or too fast. Take the time to recover.

Fatigue can be cumulative, building up over weeks. Chronic or intense fatigue can't be good. Be patient.

Heart rate can be a rough tool for monitoring work effort, fatigue level, recovery, and illness. When sitting, many people take their resting pulse rate occasionally during the day to get an idea of an average pulse rate. To find the best baseline rate, take your pulse rate when the alarm goes off in the morning before you leave bed. One caveat is that if the alarm clock frightens you every morning, lay there for a minute until your heart settles down. Take it for a minute or 30 seconds times two. Chart this every day. The rate should be consistent. If the rate is up ten beats one morning, this might be a good indicator that you are tired, having a stressful day, or that you might be coming down with an illness. As you get into better shape, the resting pulse rate usually decreases. However, everyone is different. Find out what is normal for you.

During a workout, your pulse rate will increase. The rough measure is in beats per minute (bpm). For most, the rate for intense workouts will be in the 170-180 bpm range and higher for runners in their 20s and 30s. Rates for tempo runs can approach 170-180 bpm, but no higher. Rates for long-distance runs usually range from 140-160 bpm, with it going a bit higher if you push the pace or run an extended distance. When doing interval training, which will be described later, once the rate is in the 120 bpm range between repetitions, it indicates that the person has recovered enough to start the next repetition. The older the person is, the more likely these ranges will decrease.

## RUNNING SURFACES

Spend as much time on soft surfaces as possible during your whole training cycle. Running on a soft surface instead of a hard surface will reduce the impact forces on your body from a less forgiving hard surface. There is always the caution that you need to watch the footing of the surface. Sprained ankles will set back your training. There is an element of risk/reward.

Soft surfaces like grass, chips, or dirt are great as they mitigate the impact forces on the body, especially the legs. The variety is endless and refreshing. Problems could enter the picture if the running surface is not smooth or stable, causing increased risks of twisting an ankle or knee, straining a muscle or tendon, and falling. The risk continues to climb as you become more fatigued. You want to know where your next step is going to be. If the ground is too soft, the work involved in running may rise dramatically, thus causing more significant fatigue.

A prime example would be running at the beach. This can be a real strength workout. Without gradual progression of how much running you do on it, the muscles can become overworked quickly. Extra stress would be put onto the legs if the beach is steeply slanted toward the water.

Hard surfaces are common places to run because you know where your next step will be, which is particularly important to most runners. Asphalt and cement surfaces are everywhere, most likely right out your front door. There still should be an awareness of the surface as there can be potholes in asphalt, cracks, shifting cement, and so on. On the downside, they are hard and jolt the body with more force than soft surfaces. Also, the crown of the road can bring misery, especially if there is a steep angle and the runners always run facing traffic. Be aware that on a very crowned or slanted road, this can cause changes in running gait and put stresses on the body that aren't normal.

As a reminder, you will lose if you tangle with vehicles. Be visible and pay attention to what the traffic is doing. I can't tell you the number of times I've seen people running in the dark wearing dark clothes. The next time you drive, notice how difficult it is to see people. People aren't visible unless the colors and reflective apparel jump out at you. In most cases, running on the shoulder or sidewalk facing traffic is safest so you can see oncoming traffic.

Synthetic tracks are a great place to run. They are usually softer than asphalt, so the body has less stress. You can control your pace with the exact measurement of time and distance. In many areas, an outdoor track is a safe place to run. However, the constant turns can cause stress and torque on the legs. Switch directions occasionally to balance the stress. Run in the outer lanes to diminish the stresses. If it is an indoor track, the turns are even tighter, making switching even more critical. The inside air is usually dry, which can challenge your breathing, but at least there is no snow, wind, or ice. Having exact measurements running on a track can be a great tool and stressful at the same time. Repeatedly going around the same oval can be boring as well.

Treadmills are an excellent alternative to running outside in harsh weather. If you increase the grade to 1–1.5%, you can more closely match the effort it takes to run outside. The most significant difficulties are boredom and the belt constantly moving, meaning there must be some level of concentration, or you will fly off the back.

Andre Hoeschel
UD athlete 1981–1985
5K for Bruce T-shirt
1983

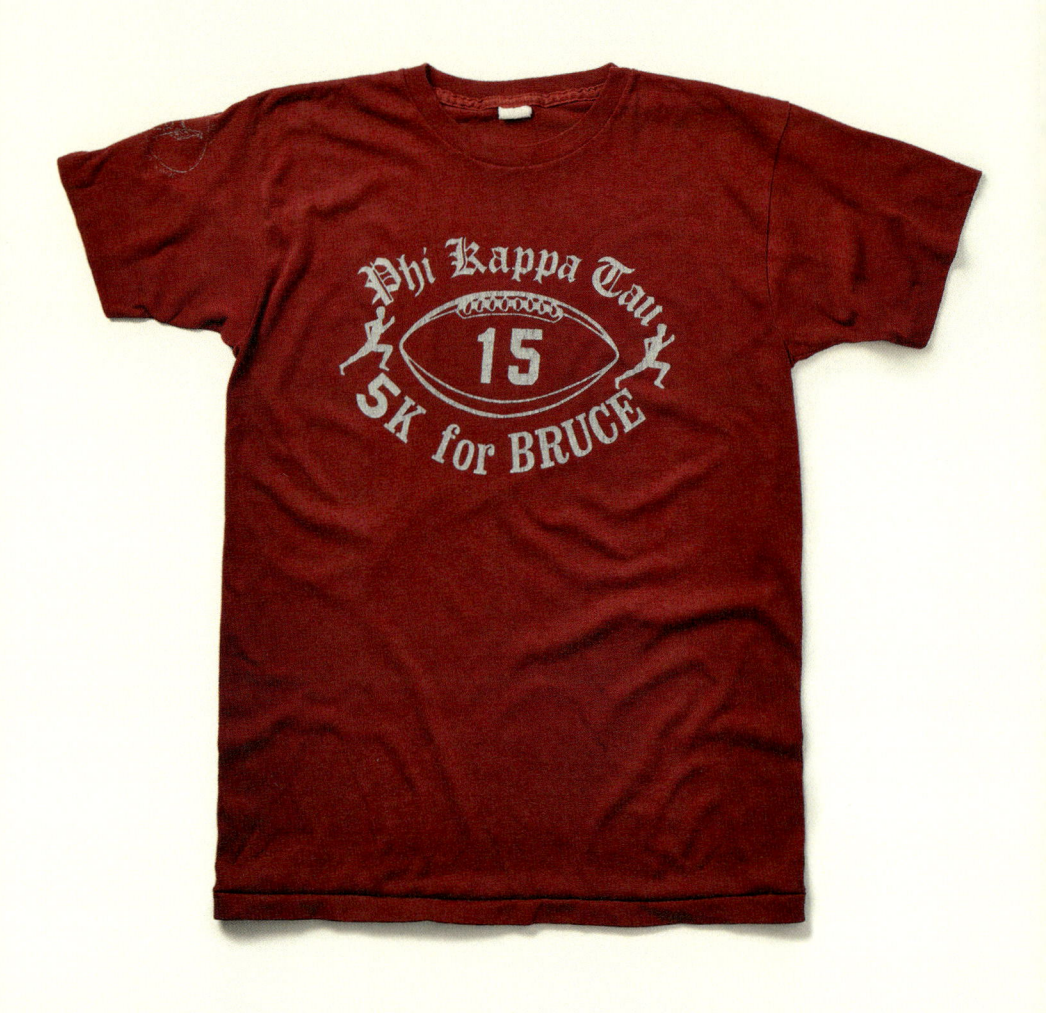

# Blessings from Running

**ANDRE HOESCHEL**

What running gave to me is very plentiful in many different ways. My biggest blessing from being a runner was helping others—specifically my former high school teammate Bruce and several other persons or charitable groups. One day during freshman year, I was out for a run. Bruce, a year behind me, still in high school, was paralyzed playing football the prior Saturday. On this run, I started thinking about what I could do to help him and his family. Being a runner, I thought maybe a 5k fundraiser race. With the help of my fraternity brothers and many others, we did it. We started the "5k for Bruce". We donated proceeds from The "5K for Bruce" race, which I started in an effort to help him and his family with certain expenses to make his life a little bit better and somewhat easier. I have the original race shirt and a few others. Also, I have the results of the 3rd race in 1985, which I think to this day was the fastest 5k Road race ever in Delaware. A time of 14.38 didn't win it. Also, there were about 25 or so runners under 17 minutes. As you know, nowadays, a sub-17 wins almost any 5k race. We also had about 1200 runners and a 14-keg post-race party later that night. Great memories, for sure!

## LIFESTYLE

Live a healthy lifestyle.

Stay hydrated. Fluids need to be taken in regularly throughout the day. This is important for the average person. Much more is required for athletes who lose significantly more fluids during activity. If you are thirsty, you are already dehydrated. Dehydration causes the blood to thicken. It lowers the blood volume, so there is less blood to circulate, making it sluggish and harder to move. This inhibits the body's cooling, affects the delivery of nutrients to cells, and delays the ridding of waste products. Signs of dehydration are feeling thirsty, dark urine color (especially in the morning), smelly clothes and sweat, dizziness, chronic fatigue, and an acute decline in body weight. An additional health issue that has affected me is that I've been bothered by kidney stones, and one of the prime factors in the formation of stones is dehydration.

There is a place for water and sports drinks in your diet. Sports drinks usually contain electrolytes and carbohydrates. While those nutrients are essential, more isn't always better. As a general rule, activities under 60 minutes in duration don't require the consumption of sports drinks in combination with a healthy diet. However, you may want something on hand during hot summer days. Besides water, sports drinks, and other liquids, great sources of fluids and electrolytes are fruits and melons. Alcoholic beverages, while liquids are generally considered dehydrating, aren't recommended. Caffeinated beverages also are considered to be dehydrating.

Hyponatremia is a condition where sodium in your system is low. The cause is often drinking too much water, which can dilute the sodium levels in the blood. People running or working out for an extended period while drinking an excessive amount of water but not replacing the salts they are sweating can put themselves in serious jeopardy of a life-threatening event because of chemical imbalances in the body. Sports drinks and average salt intake in a healthy diet can help to prevent this condition. Avoiding dehydration is essential from a performance and health perspective. Still, the message should never be "drink as much water as you can" since this can cause hyponatremia in some people.

Ensure you have proper rest, recovery, and sleep, all of which are important. When you are training, eight hours of sleep, a luxury for most, will go a long way toward better performance.

Poor eating habits can compromise both your training and race performances. Almost all of us have some diet limitations where our food affects us negatively. If you didn't have those limitations, eating fruits and vegetables, whole grains, lean meats or vegetarian options, and healthy fats such as nuts, seeds, natural peanut butter, avocados, olives, fish, and water would help keep us on top of our game. But not everyone can or likes everything. You need to mindfully determine what the best diet would be to maximize the outcomes we all desire.

Eat a colorful plate, including fruits and vegetables. An average individual should have at least five cups of fruits and veggies daily, preferably nine. Athletes should have those numbers as a minimum. The fruits and veggies should fill half of your dinner plate. This will help to ensure a large variety of essential nutrients. Salts such as sodium and potassium are necessary for chemical balance and maintaining the body's water level. Calcium is required for the bones and proper muscle functioning. Iron for the blood supply is essential.

Think balance, choice, and variety to help encourage a healthy, well-rounded diet. The body will store the extra nutrients for use at another time. Carbohydrates like fruits, vegetables, bread, cereals, grains, and honey are the primary fuel source, yielding four calories per gram of energy. These sugars and starches are good energy and are quickly and easily utilized. They can also be used during prolonged endurance efforts. Fats like meat, nuts, oils, and whole milk are another fuel source with a yield of nine calories per gram, more than twice as many calories per gram as carbohydrates, but are less easily digested. The body usually burns them at lower exercise intensities. Proteins found in meats, fish, poultry, eggs, milk, cheese, nuts, dried beans, breads, and vegetables can also be used as fuel, yielding the same number of calories per gram as carbohydrates.

But most importantly, you need protein to repair and rebuild constantly damaged or destroyed cells. For you to get stronger, proteins are essential for improved conditioning. One other note—excess fats in food can interfere with protein absorption rate.

When you restrict your carbohydrate and fat intake while engaging in intense training or limit your protein intake, an ongoing struggle arises between meeting your energy needs and essential rebuilding processes. This usually doesn't end well and may lead to injuries and overtraining.

Continued overconsumption of any nutrient groups could increase the likelihood of added stress on bones, joints, and muscles. When you eat in excess, extra calories are stored as fat, which doesn't contribute toward the energy production needed for running. This can lead to weight gain, which can add to joint stress. That doesn't mean you want to overemphasize the number on the scale, as that number can fluctuate daily, weekly, monthly, and seasonally. However, it does mean that your mind and body will benefit from being aware of your weight within the bounds of good nutrition.

Pay attention to how your system reacts to what you eat and when. Some can eat minutes before a race or workout, and some need hours ingesting only specific foods for a good result. Some might have to wait a long time after a hard effort, while others can finish and eat right away. This is something that you must figure out on your own. Don't wait until the day of a big race!

Following a tough workout or race, consume carbohydrates and some protein within 15 to 30 minutes to aid recovery. The body will assimilate the food rapidly soon after the workout or race. The rate of absorption slowly diminishes from that point forward after the activity. The rate is also slowed if a drink has too much sugar. Numerous articles recommend 80-100 grams of carbohydrate to 20-25 grams of protein, a ratio of four grams of carbohydrate to one gram of protein. Easy examples might be peanut butter and banana, a peanut butter and jelly sandwich, or a nutrition bar or snack with the correct ratio.

I've always maintained a rule discouraging the sharing of drinks to prevent the spread of illnesses. Sharing a drink from a cup or a water bottle is a nice gesture but a recipe for disaster. When cups are used, I always remind athletes to put them directly into a bag or throw them on the ground to be picked up later. I want everyone to avoid picking up a half-filled cup, thinking it was theirs while not knowing. After a workout or a race, we are all more vulnerable to succumbing to illness.

# One of the Most Popular Race Shirts Ever!

**JANET AND ED DAVENPORT**

When my brother, Jim Fischer, was coaching at Cooper High School in the Robbinsdale, Minnesota, school district, he wanted a summer fun run event for his runners. My husband, Ed, owned and managed a musical instrument repair business called Davenport Instrument Repair, and he offered to sponsor an event. So, Jim did all of the preparations, and we had one of our artist friends make up the cute T-shirt to give out to the runners. (I actually ran in the fun run, but of the four siblings in our family, I have always been the worst runner, even with my dedicated runner brothers!). We were talked into sponsoring the event for a second year. The most interesting part of the story, however, was that the T-shirts were extremely popular, and many ran the second race just to get one!

Janet and Ed Davenport
Davenport Instrument Repair
Summer Fun Run T-shirt
1970s

RUN. TRAIN. RACE.

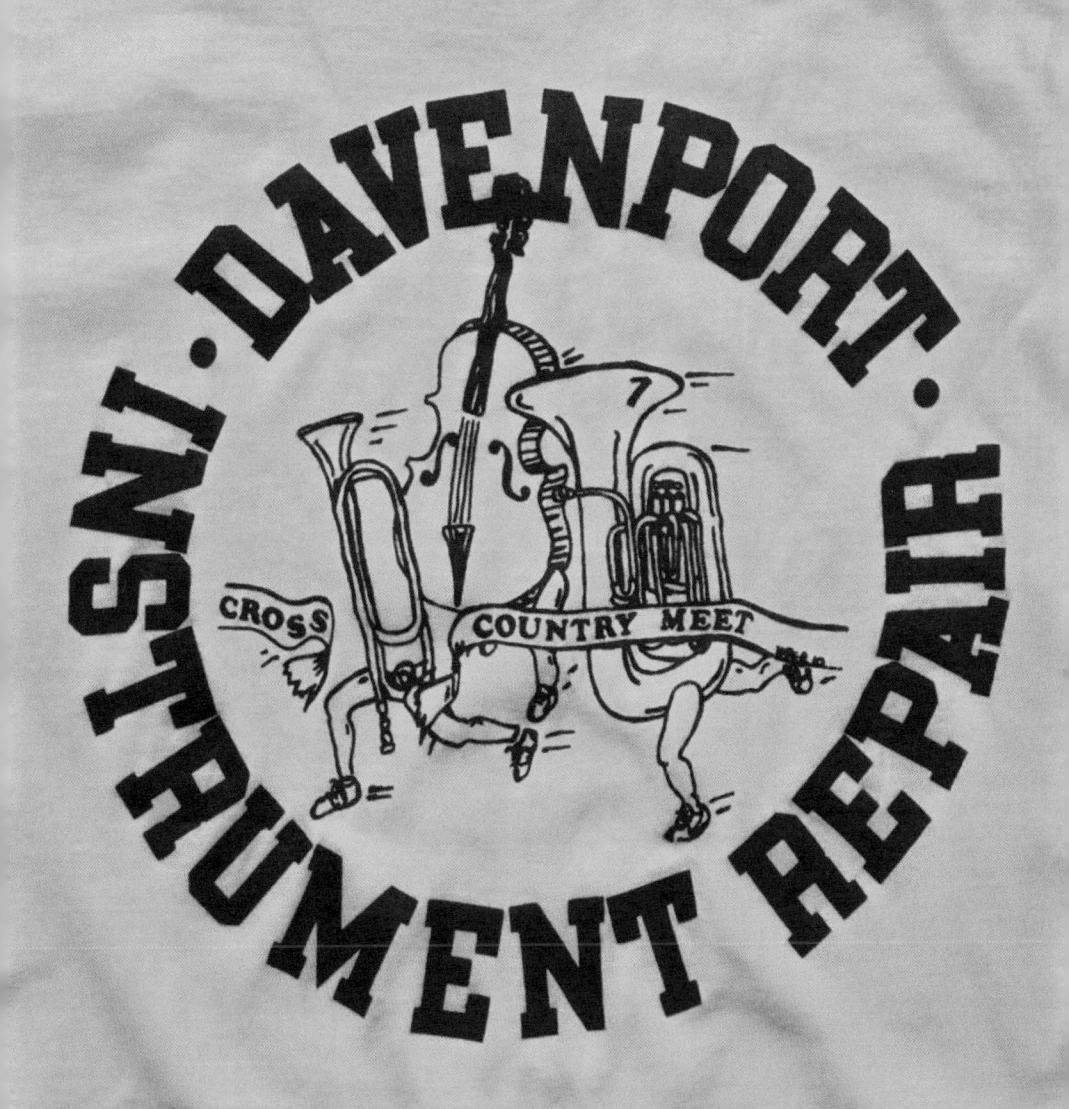

## ENVIRONMENT

Weather extremes, both mid-summer and mid-winter, zap the body of energy. In high heat and humidity, you can be hot simply standing still. Any activity will cause your core temperature to increase with sweat dripping rather than the cooling of evaporation. Under very cold conditions, it is a struggle to stay warm enough. With footing and traction issues, there are questions if you can run hard enough to keep your core temperature up. In all cases, ensure that you get enough rest and a proper diet. It generally takes upward of two weeks to acclimatize to weather changes.

## HEAT AND HUMIDITY

Heat and humidity cause problems for many. Try these suggestions to help get you through:

- Run in the cooler part of the day—early morning or late at night.
- Run in a shady area.
- Wear light-colored, lightweight, breathable clothing.
- Wear sunscreen.
- Drink cold fluids, including water and sports drinks, before, during, and after running to cool you from the inside.
- Take regular walking breaks during the run.
- Start slowly, run slower than usual, and do a shorter run.
- Break up mileage into two runs.
- Try using a treadmill or cross-train inside.
- Check your weight regularly to help monitor hydration before and after your run. Pre-run weight and post-run weight after hydration should be similar.
- Add melons to a healthy diet.
- Remember that alcohol can dehydrate you.
- Pre-cool and post-cool your body. Use an ice vest or an iced T-shirt, go to a cool room, jump in a lake, take a cool shower, sit in a cold whirlpool under supervision, or put cold packs on your head, back of the neck, armpits, and groin.
- Stop if you begin to struggle (don't let it get that far). This is another reason to take your cell phone with you.

## COLD AND WET

Winter running excuses—I grew up in Minnesota. I think that takes care of all those excuses. Exercising in the cold can help make a long winter more tolerable. Here are a few suggestions for cold weather:

- Layer up and cover up.
- Do an activity inside to raise the body temperature before going outside.
- Run for five minutes with the wind to warm up before turning back into the wind.
- Skin that is exposed can get frostbite. Cover extremities, especially the head, fingers, toes, ears, and nose, where blood supply is limited. As you get colder and colder, the body shunts the blood to the major organs, thus restricting blood flow to the extremities.
- The cold, dry air you breathe in is usually warm and humidified when it reaches your lungs. If you are concerned about running directly into the wind on a frigid day, which can be breathtaking, cover your mouth and nose with a bandana or ski mask to help warm the air. In brutally cold weather, stay inside.
- Stopping or sitting on the ground for an extended period can rapidly induce a chill.
- Wear layers of mittens and an outside wind-block layer.
- Use de-fogging products if you wear glasses.
- Traction can be a challenge. Slow down, shorten your stride, run on the gritty surface, don't make dramatic turns, limit your toe push-off, widen your base, and wear shoes or clamps for slippery surfaces. Icy conditions are a good reason to stay indoors.
- Make sure to change out of wet clothes as soon as possible. Hypothermia can be a real concern.

Cold air usually is dry, so that can promote dehydration. In extremely cold weather, the air is very dry, dramatically affecting the moisture in the lining of the respiratory system.

Layering is vital in cool or cold weather. You will usually warm up quickly if you start a little cool. You can take layer after layer of clothing off if you are too hot. You can freeze amazingly fast if you get cold while wearing minimal clothing or without layering. Heavy clothes that brace against the cold and are wet are much worse than lighter clothing that's dry. There are limits whereby cold is cold, no matter how dry you are. Wear dry clothes during low-intensity activities or other delays or breaks when recovering between repetitions or following a race. In all cases, cold, wet, and windy are a bad combination. Get out of wet clothes, including undergarments, quickly. Don't get chilled!

Manage the wind as best you can. Regarding effort, I've always felt that running into the wind hurt more than the wind at my back helped. Running into the wind always took so much effort, and I rarely felt that I was being lifted and pushed to any great extent when running with it. Don't get me wrong. Strength can be gained running into the wind, while the increased turnover running with the wind can help teach you to quicken the normal training rhythm. I'm always looking for that little extra. I've also found that after running into the wind and the intensity is high, when turning to run with the wind, keeping that same intensity, along with any benefit from the wind pushing you, will result in a naturally faster pace.

Usually, running into the wind is cooling. Runners heat up going with the wind. In the summer, run with the wind first so when you turn around, you can use the wind like an air conditioner to cool you later in the run when you are hot and tired. In the winter, go into the wind first on an out-and-back run. It will be cold. But, if you run with the wind first, building up a sweat, you will freeze when you turn back into the wind. Or you could drive out or take mass transit into the wind and run back. You will probably be peeling clothes as you go along. Tie the layers of clothes around your waist so you have them when you stop or if the wind shifts. I remember running long runs with the wind at my back in sub-zero weather, shedding clothes the whole way. Forests can also provide shelter and help block the wind.

Rain can be a big nuisance—wet hair, wet clothes, wet socks, wet shoes—heavy, sloshy, uncomfortable. At the same time, I've had some of my best and most fun workouts in the rain. Warm rain is much better than cold rain. Assess the possibilities and your attire to help determine what you should do. If lightning storms develop, all activities should be postponed. When you are done, get out of your wet clothes quickly. Again, don't get chilled!

Altitude training can prove to be a valuable tool. Adjusting to the reduced oxygen levels at higher altitudes can be a sudden challenge during the initial days, impacting your ability to perform even routine daily tasks. Teaching the body to do routine activities using less oxygen is training. Unless you live up high or plan on spending weeks there, the effect of a few days at 5,000 feet or higher may not be significant. But the theory is sound—learn to run and recover in "thin air," so fatigue starts at a higher exercise performance level when you return to a lower altitude. You may not be able to do the same amount and quality of work you need to do right away, and this is a limiting factor. It can be difficult to do high-level training and could require living at a higher altitude while going down the mountain to train at lower levels more effectively. Another issue is that the air is usually drier, magnifying dehydration.

# A Rewarding Adventure

**STEVE PLASENCIA**

Jim Fischer was my first running coach as a high schooler. Initially, I had a skeptical attitude toward running that predictably changed when I realized I was pretty good at it. Strong lungs and a competitive nature were helpful. Obstacles included a pair of very flat feet and bowed legs.

"Fisch", new to coaching in 1972, brought a calm and supportive nature. He guided me through numerous successes interspersed with untimely injuries. Our three-year efforts were fully rewarded in my final high school race, a victory in the mile at the Minnesota State High School Mile Championship.

My long running journey continued into my early 40s. Over time, I earned spots on two US Olympic Teams (1988 & 1992), four US World Championship teams, and many international competitions. As a high schooler, I never envisioned racing in over 25 countries on six continents. This international experience, the people I met, and the confidence successes built I count as the greatest rewards from my adventure. Thank you, Coach, for coaxing me into running years ago.

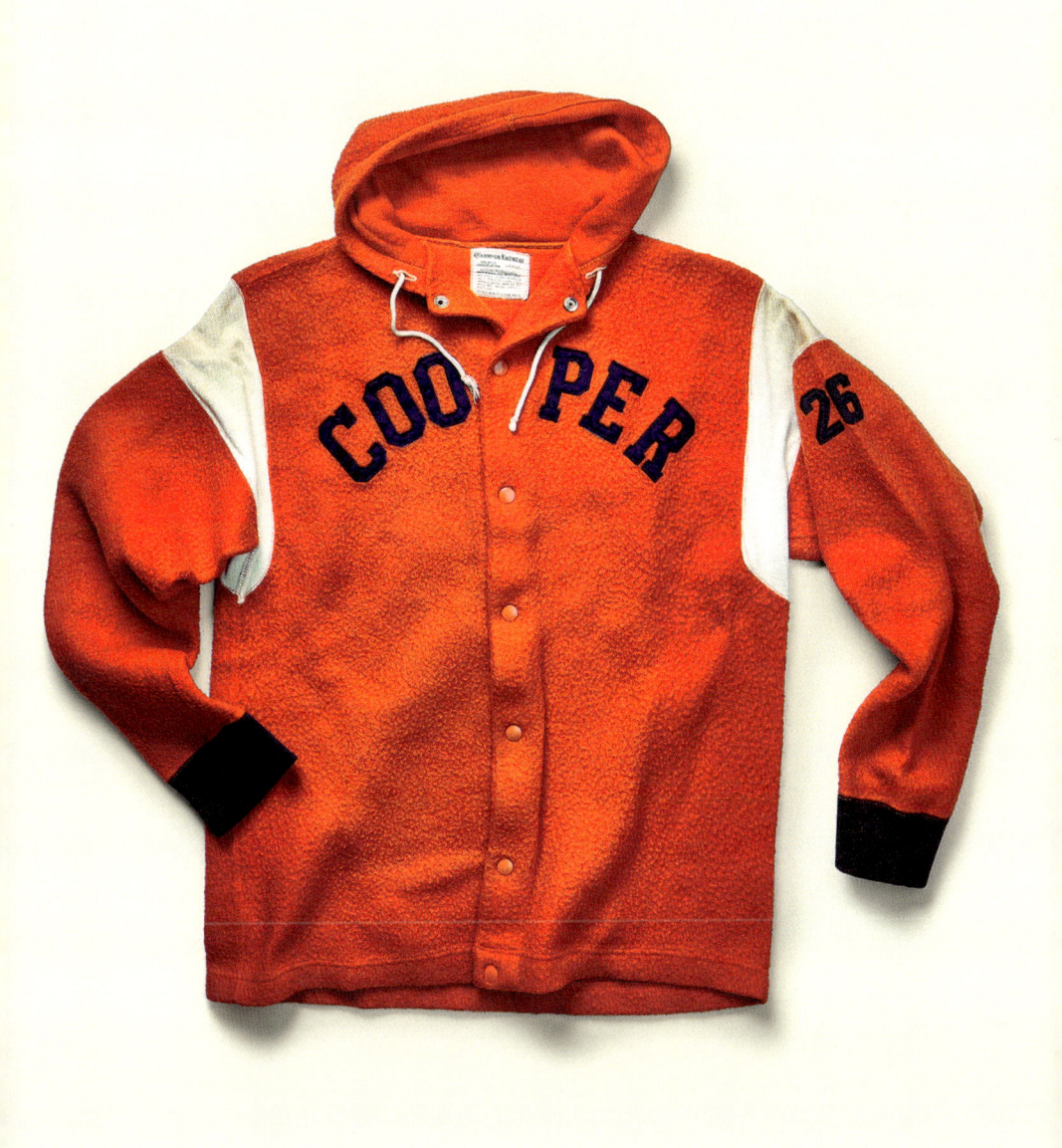

**Steve Plasencia**
**Two-time Olympian and former**
**University of Minnesota Coach**
**Cooper HS meet day**
**warmup top, 1974**

**RUN.** TRAIN. RACE.

## INJURIES

Injuries occur at some point for almost everyone. Treatment never happens quickly enough. Obviously, most are leg-related, and most of them deal with the knee or below. Professionals who deal with athletic injuries—orthopedic doctors, sports medicine doctors, physical therapists, podiatrists, and trainers who know the forces and conditions that cause the problems—are the best to diagnose and prescribe treatment to get you back into action quickly. There may be a lag time from the onset of an injury to your first appointment. Hopefully, you can get some recommendations from professionals on anti-inflammatories, pain medications, strengthening, and flexibility exercises. In the case of leg injuries, if you try to run through them, make sure you don't compensate, trying to protect the injured leg by making the other leg do more work. This can cause problems for the good leg. When coming back from an injury, don't limp or compensate. If it hurts to run, jog. If it hurts to jog, walk. If walking hurts, cross-train or rest until you can be active without pain.

I've had many injuries. I've had various kinds of knee pain: on the outside of the knee caused by a tight IT Band and weak muscles, another under the patella caused by tracking issues and muscle imbalance, another caused by cartilage issues, and still, another just below the patella caused by weak quad muscles. I've had chronic Achilles tendon pain caused by tightness I partially treated during my daily shaving time, standing on a slant board to stretch the lower leg, and standing with toes straight ahead or pointed slightly in. Once, I developed extreme pain in the outer metatarsal of my foot from the pounding following a marathon. I immediately wanted to cushion the area and protect it while, instead, building a solid arch support to take pressure off the outside part of the foot was called for. There are common sense aids or helpers that can be used to relieve causes and symptoms. Most people don't want to go to the doctor for every ache and pain. They try to ignore the pain, thinking and hoping it will disappear. Runners are notorious self-medicators with limited knowledge of the proper diagnosis or therapy. Severe pain should always be seen by a professional as soon as possible.

Strains, especially hamstring strains, need manipulation and massage to break up adhesions and scar tissue, to bring blood flow to the area, and to realign the muscle fibers. Stretching and modalities are important, but deep tissue work needs to be part of the solution.

Exercise caution to avoid stretching the injured area, as doing so may risk pulling apart the newly forming tissue. Styrofoam rollers can help to massage knotted muscles. Massage therapy can take care of tightness. Many injuries need PRICE: they need to be Protected, allowed to Rest, have Ice applied to reduce inflammation, put Compression on the area to give support, and Elevate the injury to control the inflammation. Ice initially will reduce inflammation and decrease blood flow, followed by a protective reinfusion of blood. After 24 hours, a combination of heat and ice can be used.

Sometimes, the injury is caused by something happening somewhere else in the body. A sports medicine doctor once told me to think of the back side of the body, from the base of the skull to the ball of the foot, as one piece. If there is a tightness somewhere, it could show up anywhere along that chain.

I've compiled a list of the most common running injuries and some causes, and physical therapist Andrew "Rudy" Rudawsky suggested a few things you can do while waiting for an appointment. This information can be used early in the injury process. Remember, similar symptoms might be caused by opposing issues, depending on your particular deficits. When the injury persists or affects proper mechanics, seek medical intervention.

| INJURY | SIGNS AND CAUSES |
| --- | --- |
| **Achilles Tendonitis** | Lack of flexibility, tightness, swelling, stiff shoes, speed and hill work, many miles |
| **Black Toenails** | Shoe too short, downhills, big rocks |
| **Bloody Nipples** | Rough surfaced singlet, long runs |
| **Calf Strain** | Pain and tightness in calf, intense activity, improper warmup |
| **Foot Pain (outside)** | Contusion of tendons and bones, improper alignment, lack of support, old shoes |
| **Foot Pain (top)** | Shoes tied too tight, intense or prolonged running, wrong shoe |
| **Hamstring Strain** | Extremely intense workout, overuse, dehydration, too many lunges |
| **IT Band Syndrome** | Overuse, weak quads, weak core, tight lateral hip, lack of flexibility, poor foot alignment |
| **Knee Pain** | Patellar pain, poor patellar tracking, weak quads, lack of flexibility, intense activity, old shoes |
| **Neuroma** | Narrow/tight shoes, poor shoe choices, worn-out shoes, constant contact with hard surfaces |
| **Osgood-Schlatter Syndrome** | Pain below knee, weak or tight quads, intense activity, adolescents in growth phase |

## TREATMENT

Rest, massage, rollers, stretch the surrounding area, slant board, arch supports, two-foot heel raises followed by one-foot eccentric heel lowering, strengthening, ice

Check shoe fit, bandages, ice water immersion, stay away from downhills

Band-Aids®, body gel or Vaseline®, smooth material

Rest, ice immersion, massage, flexibility, stretch surrounding area, strengthen, proper warmup, proper alignment, and mechanics

Rest, ice, arch supports, new shoes

Rest, foam protecting top of foot, modify lacing, ice immersion

Rest, ice massage, single-leg RDLs, hydrate, deep soft tissue work, stretch surrounding area including lower back, rolling, stimulation

Rest, ice stretch, massage, rolling, strengthen core, lateral hip, and quads

Rest, ice, massage, tone quads with straight-leg leg raisers (3 positions), squats and lunges, quad strength, cross-train with biking

Rest, ice, metatarsal pads, wider/better fitting shoes

Rest, ice, massage, strengthen and stretch quads

| INJURY | SIGNS AND CAUSES |
|---|---|
| **Patellar Tendonitis** | Pain below patella, weak quads, poor patellar tracking, intense activity |
| **Piriformis Syndrome** | Overuse, lack of hip flexibility and range of motion, poor posture, sleeping, and sitting positions |
| **Plantar Fasciitis** | Pain in first movements in morning or after sitting, very tight, in the foot and calf, lack of flexibility and soft tissue mobility, poor strength, flat shoes or flip flops with poor support, poor foot alignment |
| **Sciatic Nerve Pain** | Lack of flexibility and full trunk range of motion, poor posture, hip and core weakness |
| **Sever's Syndrome** | Heel pain in adolescents, swelling, redness, tightness in ligaments and tendons, tenderness when area is squeezed, trouble walking, especially in hard, stiff shoes |
| **Shin Splints** | Lower leg and foot malalignment, impact forces, hard surfaces, weak shin muscles, lack of calf flexibility, old shoes, bony stress reaction, possible fracture |
| **Side Stitches** | Muscle/diaphragm spasm, too intense too soon, overwork, poor breathing habits, wrong food, dehydration |
| **Stress Fracture** | Overuse, increased volume and/or intensity too quickly, poor shoes, hard surfaces |
| **Twisted Ankle** | Uneven surfaces, roots, poor shoes, poor balance, weak ankles and lateral hips |

## TREATMENT

Rest, ice, cross-friction massage, strengthen quads, stretch quads, patellar strapping

Ice, deep massage, stretching, strengthen core and lateral hip, correct standing, sitting, sleeping posture, improve hip range of motion

Rest, ice immersion, kneeling with toes bent forward foot stretch, calf stretch/toe raisers, slant board, foot roller, towel curls, arch support, balance pods and exercises, proper shoes

Rest, ice, deep massage, low back stretches, hip and core strengthening

Rest and/or limit activity, ice, shoes with support, inserts, massage, stretching and strengthening, avoid hard surfaces, gradually increase activity

Rest, ice massage, new shoes, shoe support and cushioning, soft surfaces, flexibility work from lower back and below, strengthen core, quads, and shin muscles, slant board, cross-train

Slow down or stop, stretch side and abdomen, massage area, hydrate, learn to belly/yoga breathe

Rest, cross-train if possible

Rest, ice, support, wrap, improve balance and lower extremity strength

# Running is more than a physical sport. It's a mental sport as well.

Laini McGonigle
Ursuline Academy Athlete
2016-2021

## ILLNESSES

Illnesses affect almost everyone at some point during the year. Take care of your diet, hydration, sleep, vaccinations, and hygiene. Avoid sharing towels, bottles, cups, and clothes, and stay away from others who are sick.

Simple handshakes, as well as dirty clothes and linens, can cause problems. Exhaustive training and racing suppress and compromise the immune system. The white blood cell count can decrease by up to 50% following strenuous activity. Athletes training strenuously are two to three times more susceptible to upper respiratory infections.

If you become sick, whether it is bronchitis, a cold, the flu, a headache, sinus trouble, or something else, you should check in with a doctor, give yourself time to recover, and start back slowly when you are healthy. For years, my athletes and I would keep running right through an illness. We would slow down a little, but that was as far as we would go. Most times, we extended the length of the illness. Over time, I saw the advantages and evidence that taking time off, getting better, and gradually getting back to training was a much better way to do things.

Ordinary people "feel good" isn't the same as working out "feel good." Walking down the street is a lot different than doing a hard workout. If you return to training after an illness, you may feel great doing a hard workout for the first ten minutes. Then, suddenly, it is like someone turned off a switch. Things can come crashing down in a hurry. You don't want a relapse, which would drag things out longer. The first few days should be easy shakeouts to see how things go. If everything goes well, ramp it up a bit. If you're dealing with an upset stomach, make a good decision about whether you can run. If it is related to the timing of your eating before running or what you had to eat, try to figure that out so it doesn't happen in the future.

With most distance runners, a sports medicine physician should check iron levels periodically for low levels, which can destroy training. Supplements and vitamins may help maintain healthy levels of iron and vitamin C.

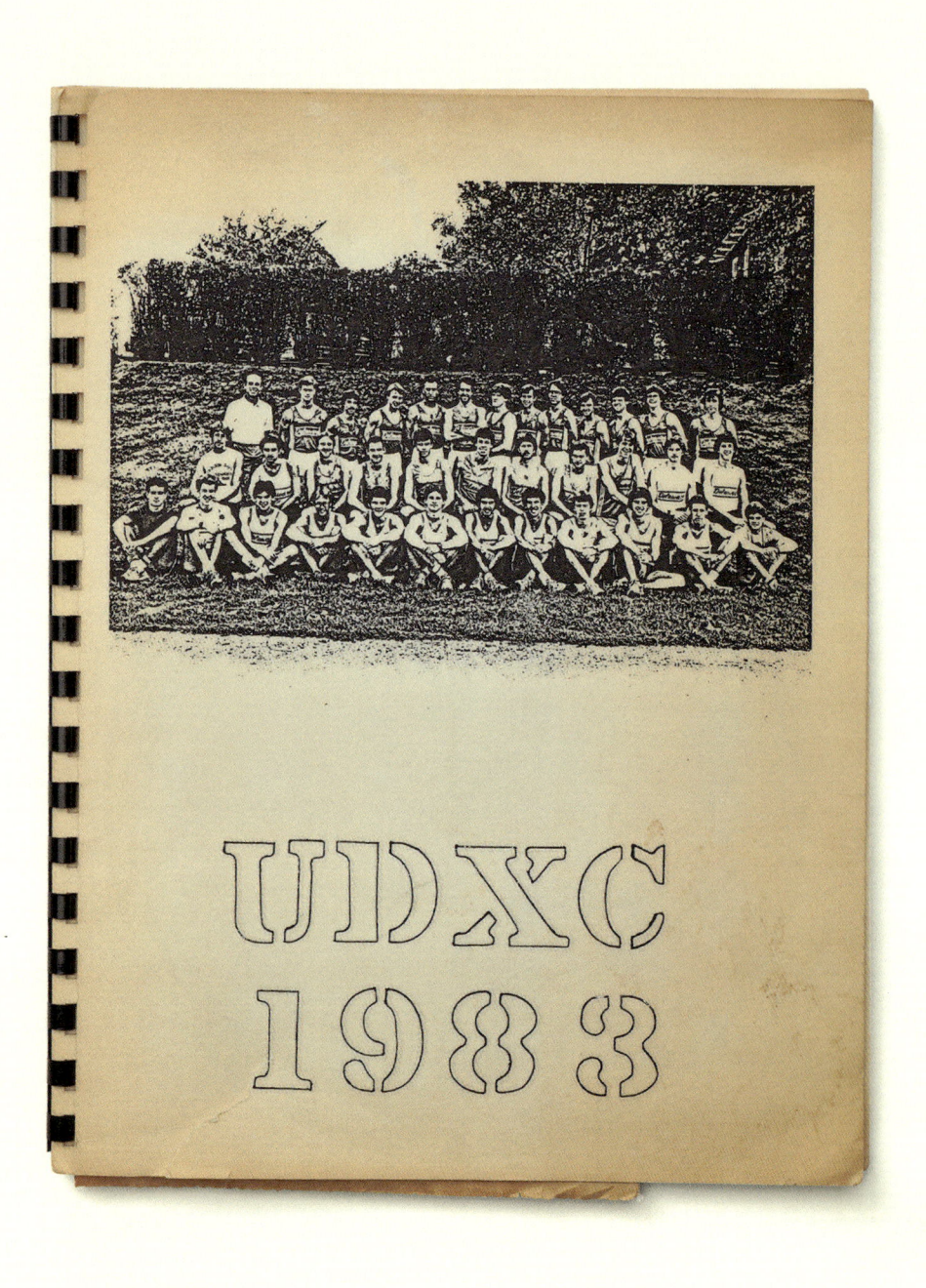

Bill Lafferty
UD athlete 1981–1985
UDXC yearly summary
booklet, 1983

# Lessons in Leadership

**BILL LAFFERTY**

As a member of the Men's UDXC and Track teams, I learned from my fellow student-athletes and coaches about the dedication, determination, and work ethic necessary to be the best student-athlete (and person) I could be. I also learned about teamwork, camaraderie, and I developed friendships that will last my lifetime. When I graduated from the University, I took those lessons learned as a student-athlete with me, and I have applied them on a daily basis in my life. More than any class that I took as a student at the University, the lessons that I learned and the qualities that I developed as an athlete best prepared me to succeed in my future endeavors.

Of course, I do not believe that my experience is unique. Indeed, I recently read an article that suggested that the number one predictor of success in law school was not a student's LSAT score; rather, the number one predictor of success in law school was whether or not the student participated in undergraduate intercollegiate athletics.

(Excerpt from a November, 10, 2008 letter to Dr. Patrick T. Harker, President, University of Delaware)

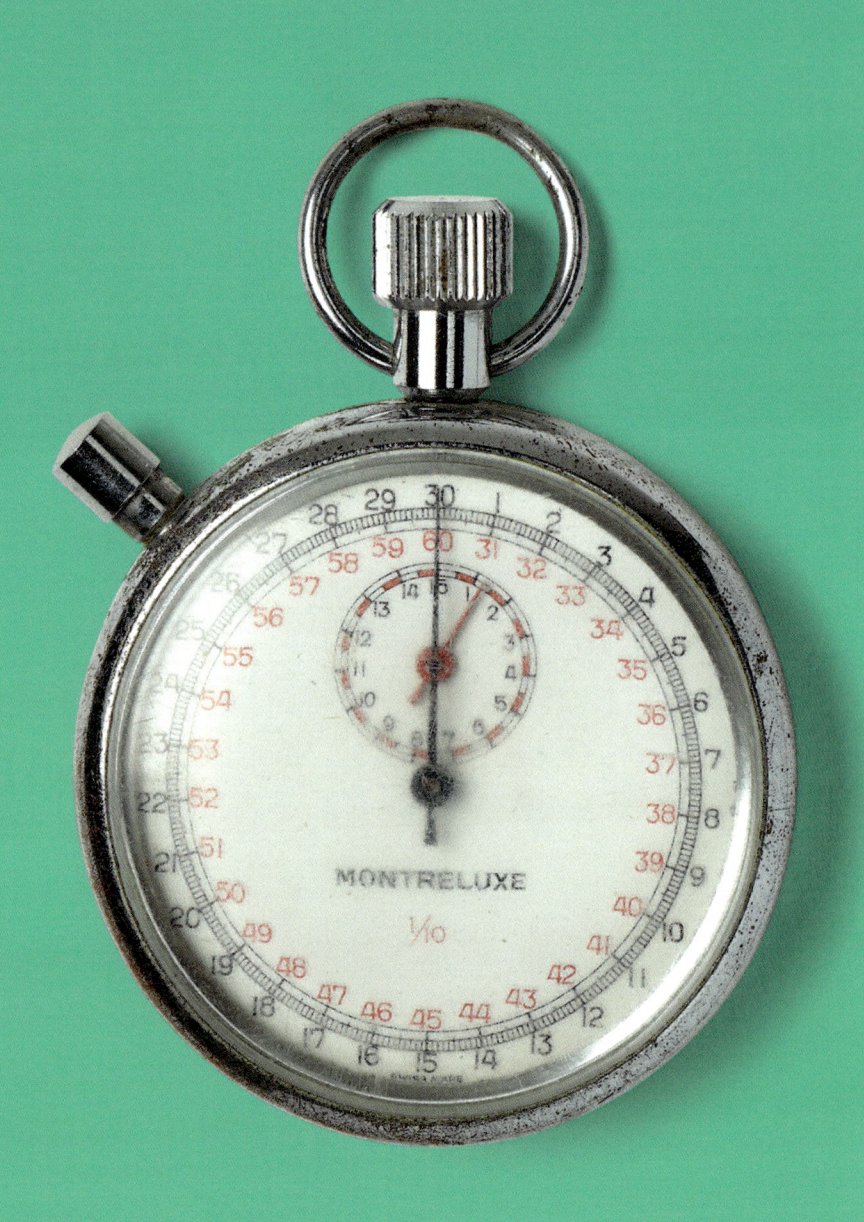

# TRAIN

I'd coached for 20+ years and had many athletes performing well. But I felt that something was missing. I called a friend, Frank Gagliano, who was at Georgetown at the time, and asked if I paid for his lunch, would he spend two hours talking about training and how he put things together. He said he certainly would, as he had no secrets. After two hours, so many light bulbs went off that I couldn't wait to get home and write things down. The results for my team were immediate, not because of many new workouts but because, now, all the puzzle pieces were fitting. Once I learned the basics, I worked hard, fitting workouts and training together in meaningful ways.

**Jim Bray**
**UD athlete 1974-1977**
**Stopwatch**
1970-1972

## HERE ARE FIVE THINGS I WANT YOU TO JUMP START YOUR TRAINING

1. Find a coach/advisor to get you to a place you can't get to by yourself.

2. Work hard, but more and harder isn't always better. Control your training to make you stronger.

3. Recovery from good work will give the body time to strengthen between workouts.

4. If you have a weakness, the race will find it. Maximize your strengths and cover every weakness so there are no more left.

5. Be patient!!

## THE PREPARATION

Some people want a little more than exercise. They want to challenge themselves to become a little stronger, run a little faster, go a little farther, enter a race, set a personal record, qualify for an event, place in their age group, win a race, or become a person who is recognized as a top-flight racer. Some think about winning races and championships. Remember that performance and winning are outcomes. Performance comes from concentrating on doing the work and all the things needed to be at that higher level. People worry about how they'll perform rather than thinking about what they need to do to get the desired results. Everyone can improve a little or a lot, finish a race, or set a personal record. Putting in the correct training will prepare you to accomplish your goals with the feeling you are prepared and in control.

You do a workout to stress the body, so you will build yourself stronger to handle the stress and get into better shape, so you can recover faster and race at a higher level, so you can workout harder to stress the body, so you will build yourself stronger to handle the stress and get into better shape, so you can recover faster and race at a higher level, so you can workout harder to stress the body. The cycle continues…

What's the process for improvement? How do you gauge the right amount of training? These are the questions I'll address. To steer away from stagnation, I'll echo the old adage: "If you do what you always did, you'll get what you always got." Regardless of your goals, there are steps you can take to enhance your performance. You have the flexibility to decide the intensity and extent of your training.

You can control two things—your attitude and your effort. Rod Olson emphasizes these in his book *The Legacy Builder*. I've also heard preparation added to those two things. You need to develop a passion to get better. Be 100% committed, and with the resources, you must improve. Fitness is the adaptation to stress. Training manipulates duration or volume, intensity, and density to overload the system and make the body adapt. That doesn't mean that you need to max out in every workout. Live to train another day. You might be a young athlete with energy, time, and desire or a senior runner with a family and full-time job. Decide what amount of time and energy you can spend, and then determine a plan that can give the best results for your efforts.

There are some general differences to keep in mind between women and men. Men have more muscle mass. Women have a lower center of gravity. Men have a narrower pelvis. Women have narrower shoulders. Men have a larger chest. Women have a longer trunk length proportion. Men have a longer leg length proportion. Women have fewer sweat glands and begin sweating at a higher temperature. Men have a greater maximum oxygen uptake and have larger hearts. Women don't dissipate heat as well. These differences may alter the actual work that can be done or the training that needs to be done. It also changes the visual perception of what is being done.

I'll list some positive qualities I see in runners who raced for me. This is a good list. Each runner may not have all of these traits but think about which ones apply to you: ambitious, attentive, calm, cheerful, committed, confident, consistent, controlled, courageous, creative, dedicated, dependable, determined, disciplined, engaged, excited, fit, flexible, focused, healthy, helpful, instinctive, intelligent, intense, leader, listener, mentally tough, motivated, organized, pain tolerant, passionate, perseverant, persistent, positive, prepared, relentless, resilient, respected, good sports person, strong, successful, supportive, talented, trained, trusted, and hard working. If you want to be highly competitive, you want to maximize your potential. Some need to find a way to win. I understand. Not everyone has the same abilities or desires. Training should be progressive so you keep getting better and better. But, at the same time, you need to be patient and plan for the long term. During my average running career, no matter how hard I worked, there were people I wouldn't beat. Set that thought aside for a minute. Let's say that you want to plan for a best-case scenario. Let's say that you want to make a plan that will make you competitive and put you on the top of the awards stand. Now, let me give you something to think about. The puzzle is this: What must you do to beat someone in a 5K who can run a mile ten to 15 seconds faster than you can? Can you find qualities that you have that you can train to make you strong enough to overcome the talent the other person has? You may not have the qualities to overcome that talent, but you may. If you plan it well enough, can plain old hard work get you where you want to go? Let me give you an example of a question that an elite athlete might ask. An elite athlete is equal in fitness to the other competitors. Some competitors have more leg speed and can run a 400m dash much faster than the elite athlete. If everyone is together with 400m left in the race, what are the odds that the elite athlete will win? Think about what you need to do to put yourself into the conversation.

After I finished college and was at my first teaching job, I did some fitness activities but wasn't training. I was sitting in the stands at my college's homecoming football game in the early 1970s when a couple of my former teammates started talking about the marathon they would run the next day. Running a marathon had been in the back of my mind as something I wanted to accomplish on my bucket list. Of course, I told them that I would join them. The race was the City of Lakes Marathon, which led to the Twin Cities Marathon in the Minneapolis-Saint Paul area. The first half of the marathon went OK as my fitness and running background pulled me through in about 1:33. I felt good about myself then. About three miles into the second half of the marathon, things started to go south. I was a little over

Live to train another day.

an hour slower in the second half of the marathon. It wasn't a pretty sight. My muscles were cramped. My feet were very sore because of the distance and shoes I was wearing. I was in extreme pain the last few miles, trying to jog a few steps each minute between my slow, hobbled walk. With all the fitness work I'd done in high school and college, this was a huge lesson in the importance of specific preparation and training. I wanted to learn about the process to improve my coaching knowledge and running.

Find someone to help guide you, someone you can trust with your training plan: a coach. A good coach helps you get better results than you could get by yourself. This person should have your best interests in mind, be willing to give information, and help you with ideas and adjustments to make your training effective. The planning process is called periodization. This includes the planning, goals, and objectives and how to manage the biomotor abilities: speed, endurance, strength, flexibility, and coordination. We'll get to these later.

One of the first questions I get is about mileage. "How many miles should I run?" If you are starting, the focus should be on ensuring you don't do too much and don't go too fast. It would be best if you stayed comfortable with your pace and only run for a short time, a short time at that. After the initial weeks of getting used to the exercise, you can gradually increase the amount of time you run. When you are ready to start increasing your running, you can get into a training schedule. If you feel you have advanced past the beginner stage, you can step back into your schedule, gradually building to a more demanding level. People who are just starting to run and are working to increase the amount of running they are doing or are working to maintain pace while on a long run should consider taking periodic walking breaks. They can drink fluids, go to the bathroom, and give their body a little time to refresh before starting to run again. Walk before you HAVE to walk because if you get to the point where you are struggling to run another step, it is too late.

Emily (Gispert) Weaver
UD athlete 2010–2014
UDXC T-shirt and
hair ties, 2011

# Team Culture

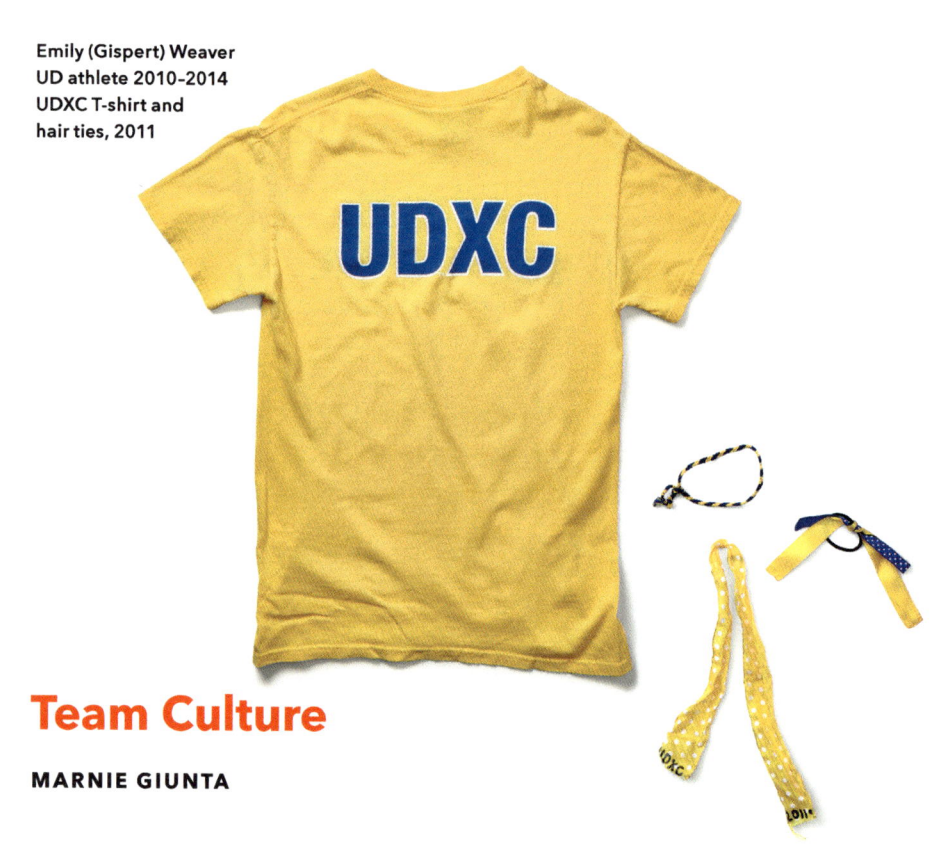

**MARNIE GIUNTA**

Coaches put extensive efforts into developing a team culture where the expectations are maintaining athletic excellence year after year. Team culture is the cornerstone in achieving success as an athlete and a coach. The pride one feels while wearing that team emblem is a significant motivational factor in the athletes' tenacious competitive efforts.

I'm a Pittsburgh native who joined the University of Delaware's (UD) Cross Country and Track & Field teams. I knew no one. On that first day of practice, we set out to run an easy five-mile run. I ran a personal best for those "easy" five miles. I returned to my dorm room, overwhelmed, thinking, "What have I gotten myself into?"

As each day passed, it got easier. It got easier because I found a friend in another teammate who felt the same way I did. It got easier because the team leaders began including me in their running group. After all, my performances were beginning to equal theirs, and they wanted to challenge me. It got a little easier because of the team dinners at Sbarro's every Friday night and the long van rides to and from meets. There were many laughs and lots of fun facts being shared. It got a little easier because I was giving/

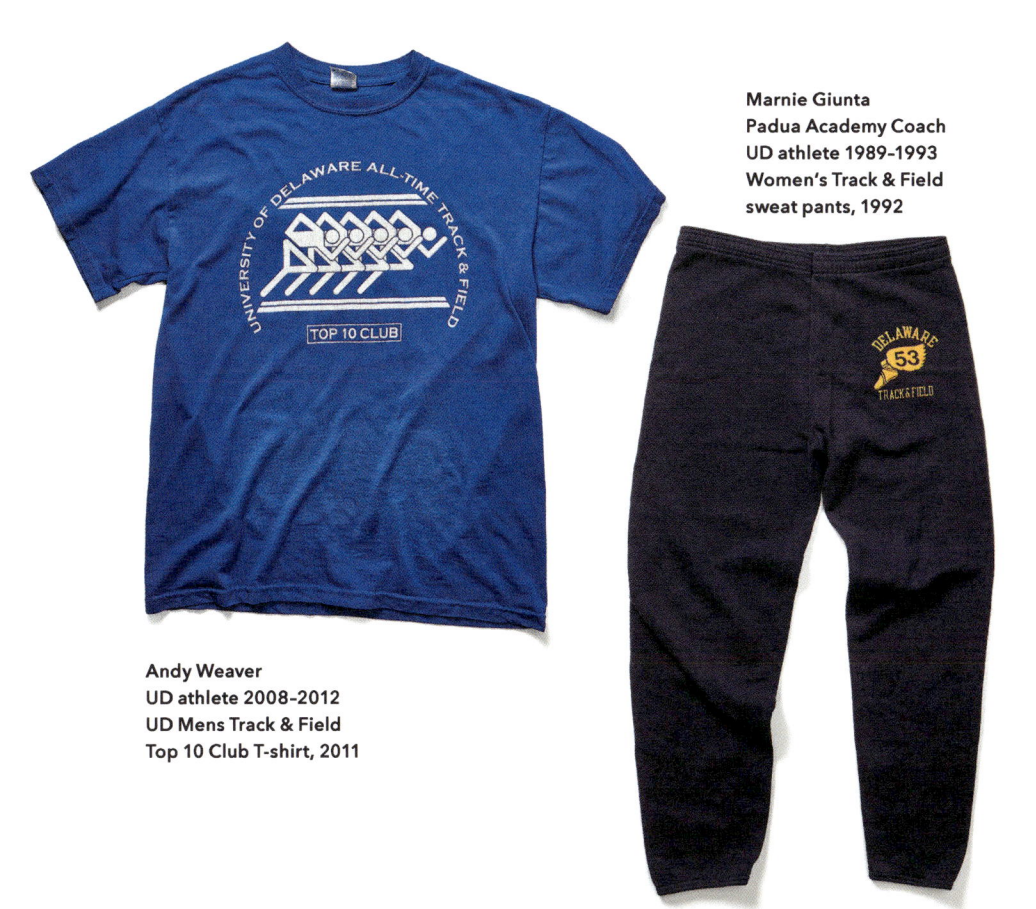

**Andy Weaver**
UD athlete 2008-2012
UD Mens Track & Field
Top 10 Club T-shirt, 2011

**Marnie Giunta**
Padua Academy Coach
UD athlete 1989-1993
Women's Track & Field
sweat pants, 1992

receiving gifts or joining teammates for celebrations at Choate Street or Papermill apartments after every meet, for birthdays, or the end of the season. It got a little easier because my teammates were, in fact, my family.

When it was my turn to lead the team, I needed to pay forward everything I experienced. I welcomed the new team members, showed them how to work, treat one another, never settle for just good, and most importantly, celebrate one another's achievements as a "family." We do this so the traditions continue. We do this so our team pride continues to be passed along.

I am so grateful for my experiences as a collegiate athlete. They helped prepare me for life's challenges, knowing that nothing is out of reach, especially with the support of "family."

I have many to thank for my successes as a runner and coach. Jim Fischer is one of those people. He's known as Coach to everyone. As I reflect on my coaching career, I know that my team's culture is modeled by my positive experiences at UD and Jim's kindness, inclusiveness, respect, and sincere belief that everyone can become a champion.

RUN. **TRAIN.** RACE.

When I was training in high school and college, I did the same workouts week after week. That can be good if you are measuring progress. For me, it was tedious. One of the main tenets of my approach is variety. It helps keep the mind and body engaged. A variety of workouts test different muscles, help maintain a good range of motion, and stress your physical, mental, or emotional capacities. This doesn't mean I ignore the need to repeat workouts to monitor progress. I use this on a limited basis.

Another thing to note is that the body responds well to change. Routines must be changed periodically to keep the nervous system fresh and excited. This also helps to avoid the feeling of becoming stale or hitting a plateau.

Training is a continuum. You start running wherever you are—slow, fast, weak, strong, small, big—and gradually get better. You need to monitor your recovery from day to day. After you are consistently running four days per week, you should consider adding another day each week, then later make one of the days a little longer and slower, then make one of those days a day of intensity, then add another mile or ten minutes to one day, then try to raise the amount of intensity on your hard day, then add another day of intensity, and so on. Gradually increase the length and intensity of your running. I'll often use the term comfortably hard when describing your intensity. Run hard, but control your effort. Make sure you have good form, and don't be sloppy. Be patient. Each step is an explosion you want to build stronger and stronger over time. You want to train smart, not simply hard!

Training is a continuum. You start running wherever you are—slow, fast, weak, strong, small, big—and gradually get better.

## TYPES OF WORKOUTS

Understand the purpose of the workouts that you do. You may find multiple ways to get the same result. Make sure you know what results you are trying to achieve and why. Identify goal race distances and plan your training accordingly. It is difficult to train for all distances at the same time. An 800m race takes approximately 50% aerobic (continuous movement fueled by oxygen from the air you breathe) work and 50% anaerobic (high-intensity movement driven by energy stored in your muscles). Racing a marathon is about 98% aerobic. It is difficult to concentrate on your training when the disparity in training necessities is so significant. That doesn't mean that you can't race well over many distances. You can develop overall fitness that will allow you to be strong any time you step to the starting line. Whatever the workout, you want to do the second half of the workout equal to or stronger than the first half so you can practice being strong at the end. More isn't always better, but not enough is almost always worse. Incorporate variety into your training specific to race efforts and race conditions such as terrain (flat, rolling, hills), surface, heat, humidity, cold, wind, altitude, and shoes.

You will put together many elements of training to achieve your goals. Below are all the possible workouts you can incorporate in your training. Later in this book are some training schedules that show how to integrate them into your program.

**Fartlek training**

This is Swedish for speed play—free form, undefined interval training. The genesis for this type of workout is a "spirited" run on trails through the forests and around the lakes, working and playing with the terrain. Run long, run short, sprint a hill, walk, do what you want to do when you want to do it. Generally, during the first half of the workout, do longer, slower segments to ensure you are thoroughly warmed up before doing higher-intensity sprints or hills. The variety of scenery takes the struggle out of the effort. Sometimes, you could play mind games like beating an unknowing person to the fork in the path, catching someone before the top of the hill, making sure that no one passes you during the run, or getting to the stop sign before being passed by ten cars. In-line single file running where, time after time, the person at the end of the line goes to the front could be a type of fartlek training.

**Hills (Uphill)**

Embrace hills. Look forward to them with an evil glint in your eyes. Racing on hills is strenuous. It can also be very technical. Practice is for training and is also for technique. Hill training involves both going up and down hills. People who run are keenly aware of going up a hill. Hills can be short, long, steep, gradual, or combined. Uphills are associated with the strength of the muscles, cardiovascular system, and mindset. Think of steep hill reps as speed-power training and long hill reps as strength-endurance training with minimal change in running form. One problem with uphill running is that it can slow the running rhythm, especially when you get near the top. This needs to be monitored so as not to slow your overall running rhythm. As with so many other types of training, this should be addressed consistently. Distance runners often work on long, more gradual hills to sustain an effort while keeping their running form close to normal. You shouldn't rule out a once or twice-a-week set of short hills to gain power and make your leg and foot action more dynamic.

There are things to consider in practice that will directly influence your racing. When approaching a hill, especially a steep hill, accelerate before you reach the hill. You will gain momentum before you begin the hill. Use good form. Don't bend at the waist when going up a hill. Your stride is already going to be shorter. Bending at the waist will shorten your stride and cause you to lose power in your push-off. This isn't efficient. You can lean into the hill, but the lean comes from your ankles, not your waist. Stay on your toes and drive your arms more forcefully, working harder to inspire your legs. Make sure to lift your toes because if you drag them, you will trip. You might take a glance or two toward the top of the hill to see where you are, especially when assessing your energy levels, but otherwise, tend to your business at hand, the ten to 20 meters directly in front of you. When climbing a hill and cresting it, don't stop or slow down at the top, but keep going ten, 20, or 30 meters past the crest of the hill. It is called "running over the top" to maintain momentum and gain some ground on the people who shut down or stop on the crest of the hill.

I'll mention this again later, but for the most part, there are two main ways to get up a hill. You can maintain your effort, which will slow down your running speed, or you can keep your running speed, increasing your effort. There are situations when you might want to do one and other times when you want to do the other. Practice them both. Are you training in an area without hills? Try running bridges, stadium steps, stairwell steps, shallow water, or soft sand. While they aren't the same, they can be a good substitute. Doing something completely different can be hard work and fun. My high school kids would travel to Memorial Stadium (since taken down) on the University of Minnesota campus and run the stadium—30 sections of stairs going up one and down the next, 62 steps each to the top, with each step getting taller as you run up. Some would get to the end, turn around, and do it in reverse. Of course, you must be careful of doing too much, but you get the picture. Even when you don't want to do hill repeats, or it isn't in the program for a specific part of the training cycle, you can stay in touch with this by doing hilly runs.

**Hills (Downhill)**

Downhill running must be practiced. Most people think that gravity will make everything easy. This should be "free money." This is indeed a "help" with your pace. The faster speeds take a lot of energy and can be exhausting. It would be best to practice on a downhill that goes down gradually, not on a steep one. To take full advantage of a downhill, you must learn to flow down the hill. Be perpendicular to the grade of the hill with minimal changes in your form. Many people running downhill have their first foot contact well in front of their bodies. This "hard heel" puts on the brakes every step and sends massive jolts and impact forces throughout the body. Braking gives you control but slows your speed and increases the impact forces. You will also probably be leaning backward, making this an even more miserable experience. That makes the downhills a hurt rather than a help. The quads in the upper leg, trying to handle all of this, can be dramatically weakened, hurting performance. Make sure to slightly bend the knees so you don't make contact with a straight leg. The bent knee acts as a stiff shock absorber. Rather than reaching the foot out in front of the body to have huge strides, bring the foot back toward the body before contact is made.

The action of the foot is like a ball rolling down the hill rather than a stiff board hitting with a hard heel and plopping down one after another. This must be practiced along with a much faster stride frequency, e.g., faster steps. Practice turnover using a low-grade downhill with a smooth, softer surface to reduce impact rather than a steep downhill. Part of the problem with downhill running, especially on trails or in cross country, is that it is much more difficult to see where you will put your foot down than when you are going uphill. You trust the surface, and sometimes that can be a faulty notion causing ankle and knee problems. You will find another thing to get used to—much quicker arm movement. It only makes sense that the arms must mirror the faster leg motion. I've found that when first practicing downhill running, some athletes hold their arms out wider, partly for balance and partly because the arms can't keep up. They lose rhythm and get out of sync. This is a significant reason for practice. As you get used to running downhill quickly, your arms come closer to your body, and it looks increasingly like normal arm motion.

**Interval training**

This is running predetermined repetitions separated by rest intervals. Hard anaerobic training increases muscular force. However, the accumulation of lactate works against the proper functioning of the mitochondrial metabolism, the power center of each muscle's cells. This training can teach the body to tolerate and dissipate lactate. It allows you to run fast in smaller segments and relies on the manipulation of five variables: the length of the repetition (time or distance), the number of repetitions, the speed of the repetitions, the length of the recovery (time or distance), and the nature of the recovery (slower run, jog, walk, stand, etc.). Overall workout factors to be considered are volume (meters), intensity (speed), and density (how close together). Depending on the workout, repetitions can be grouped into sets. This allows you to complete one group or set and take extra time to "freshen up" before starting the next group of repetitions. Doing all repetitions without taking a little more time partway through the workout would be more challenging. However, this shouldn't be done if the last part of the workout is poorly performed or is a real struggle. With regular interval training, I recommend jogging during rest periods as often as possible. The circulation to the muscle cells is greater, bringing oxygen and nutrients and clearing wastes at a higher rate. It has been said that two-thirds of the recovery occurs during the first minute of the rest period. This is an approximation—keep moving. (See Workouts on page 195–197 for examples.)

Monitor the number of meters of intensity in a workout just like you would monitor the number of miles you run per week. If you do 8 x 1000m, that's 8000m of intensity. It doesn't include the warmup, warm-down, or recovery, just the meters of intensity. This will change slightly from workout to workout and also in the different phases of your training. You want to be aware so changes are something you plan for and are not surprised by.

There are many ways to put these variables together. Variety is a great way to keep you engaged in the training process. An excellent exercise would be to take a distance, say a 1000m repetition, and think of how to make up workouts that would work at various times during the year. Early in the training cycle, the volume and number of repetitions would be high while jogging the short rest intervals and keeping the intensity low, e.g., 8 x 1000m @ 10K pace with a 200m jog recovery. As the competitive season approaches, the volume would stay the same, the rest intervals would be longer, and the intensity higher, e.g., 8 x 1000m @ 5K pace with a 400m jog recovery. As the championship or goal race season approaches, the volume would decrease, the rest intervals would increase even more, and the intensity would be high, e.g., 3–5 x 1000m @ 3K pace with 800m jog recovery. Again, try to make up workouts that would be appropriate when training for any distance race at any time of the year using a variety of repetition lengths.

The repetition length can be short, even for long-distance athletes' training. I've heard marathon runners talk of doing a workout they called 200 meters until dusk. The big issue with short reps is many don't control the pace. For most people, the speed automatically increases when the repetition is shorter. And there may be times when faster reps might be great. If you want to do a large volume of work, you can't let your control of the pace get away from you. You control the workout. Don't let the workout control you.

Another way of organizing a workout is to do cut-down sets. Cut-down means getting faster as the workout goes on. One way is where each set of reps gets progressively faster. Another is as the set proceeds, each repetition gets a little faster. The workout gets faster, no matter which way you are doing it. This is again promoting the idea of being strong when you are tired. You can get carried away with wanting to go faster and faster. Work hard, but be in control.

# A Successful Team

**ANNA PRYOR**

The coach created an encouraging and supportive team environment that strengthened our team's sisterhood. Every athlete knew their role and importance to the team. With that, we all bonded over our shared passion, drive, and determination for running. These factors made teamwork second nature. We all had one goal in mind—to be State Champions. We pushed each other and made hard work fun, because for the team success, there must also be individual success.

Three years in a row our team won the state title in cross country. This was possible because we were able to strategize and motivate each other before, during, and after our race. I feel so grateful to have been an asset on a tight knit, successful, powerful, and loving team.

Anna Pryor
Ursuline Academy
athlete 2017–2022
UAXC rugby shirt
2022

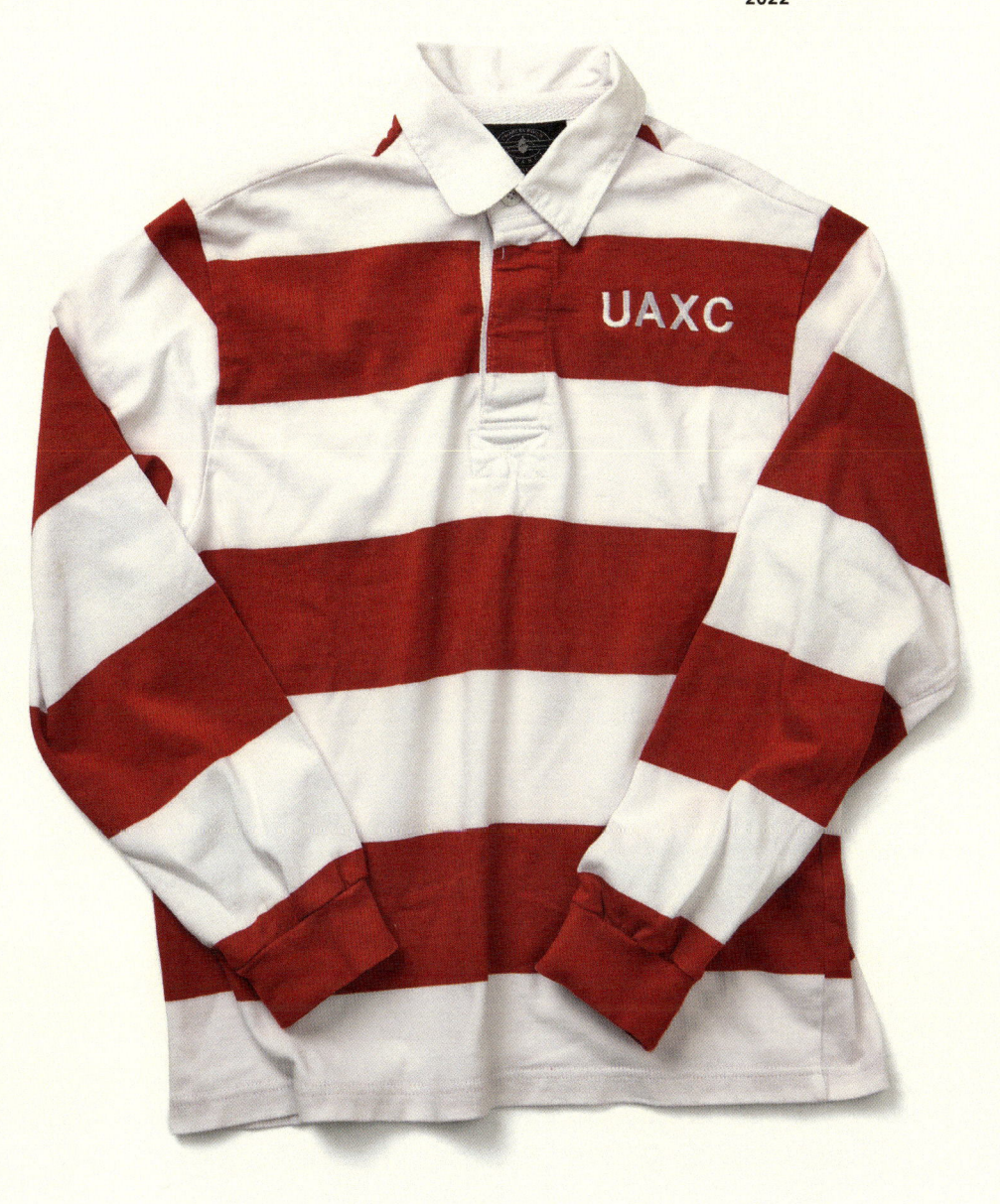

RUN. **TRAIN.** RACE.     85

I frequently use workouts I call "recover on the run." These workouts are like interval workouts, but instead of walking or jogging in between repetitions, you ease back slightly, trying to recover while you are still moving at a relatively fast pace—a float. Depending on when the workout is run during the cycle, volume, intensity, and density are important factors. Practice this concept. An example would be breaking a 600m repetition into 200m segments, running a strong 200m followed by a float 200m with a return to the pace of the first segment for the last 200m. Or, if you were doing a continuous run, you would alternate strong, and float segments the whole time. There have been times during long races when I noticed that I was on the edge of struggling. This is where "float" training comes in. I dropped my arms and shoulders, relaxed my breathing, and consciously reduced the effort of my pace. I thought that by the time I got to the next mile marker, I would have slowed by 20 to 30 seconds in that mile. My pace had often slowed by five, maybe ten seconds in that mile. It was like taking a little break while still covering ground. This can also be used as surge training. Use your imagination based on the basic principles of your training cycle and the five interval training variables.

Make sure that you practice running all the way through the finish line on every repetition. For example, an 800m rep isn't a 799m repetition or race. It is 800m long. You can lose a race on a last-second lean at the finish line, miss a record, or qualifying by a fraction of a second. Coach Roy Griak made it clear to emphasize that you should "Run ten meters past the finish line." Do it correctly in practice so that it becomes second nature, and you won't have a problem in a race. Get into the habit right away. You have done all that work. Carry it a few seconds longer.

Interval training can be done on a track, on the roads, in a park, or wherever you want. You can define the repetitions and rest periods by time or distance. There are advantages and disadvantages to either method. There may be times when you may want to know exactly how fast you are running a certain distance on the track, and there may be times when you want to "feel" your effort in a local park where you don't know the exact distance. Both have a place.

**Long distance run**

The weekly long-distance run is important. The long run will give you extended time on your legs, help you learn concentration, mental toughness, and perseverance, assist the body in learning how to utilize fats (saving carbohydrates for later), work to strengthen and increase the durability of the heart and muscle cells, make bones more resistant to injury, increase the enzymes aiding in aerobic energy production, build more mitochondria (power plants in cells), and help the body develop the capillary bed at the cellular level in the muscles. It should be done at an easy, even conversational pace. What makes the long run hard is that it is a long run. Don't make it doubly tough by running it fast unless that's the planned workout. The long run comprises about 20% to 25% of the weekly mileage, although there are training plans where it would make up a higher percentage. The long run is the slowest day of the week, maybe one to two minutes per mile slower than your regular run. But don't be sloppy with your running form. Maintain good body mechanics.

Don't start out too fast because it is going to be a long day. Keep your pace as even as you can, possibly negatively splitting (getting a little faster) the run. Everyone, depending on their fitness level, has a point at which they have maximized the "good" out of the run, and to go farther would risk injury or illness. Be conscious of fatigue levels before, during, and after the run. A run longer than two and a half to three hours may significantly increase the possibility of injury. There will be times when you will do a long run at a faster pace. That would be a workout with different objectives. During a long run, you could take short drinks or rest breaks to help refresh. This is especially important when increasing the distance of the long run. As the run gets longer, the legs must learn to function when tired. The longer the run continues, there is an increase in the ratio of fats to carbohydrates used as fuel utilized by the muscle cells. It isn't an on-off switch; carbohydrates are predominantly used for short runs and fats for long runs. Fats are used to a larger percentage as the run goes longer and longer. Typically, about two to three capillaries feed each muscle cell. The long run will help the body increase the number of capillaries feeding each cell up to eight, nine, or ten. That means the cardiovascular system can deliver food and oxygen more efficiently to the cells and remove waste. There is a point of diminishing returns—risk/reward. It varies from athlete to athlete, training schedule to training schedule. For many, three hours might be that point. For others, it may depend on the athlete.

Some feel pressure to do one long run each week even though they aren't confident. Their long runs beat them up because of weakness or weather or whatever. Try splitting the distance with one or more breaks, or try morning and evening runs to total the distance until you can do it in one session. You could try back-to-back days with moderately long runs that count more than what the single long run would total.

Long workouts can be done like a long progression run, a long race modeling workout, or a marathon simulation. They are important to the training process but usually have different purposes and functions. You may need more recovery than a normal long run.

**Marathon simulation**

This is a run at your projected marathon pace. You want to get familiar, locked in, comfortable, and confident with the pace you want to run in your goal race. I recommend building up to a 13-mile distance, but this can be longer for the more experienced athlete. You can break the run into sections, especially when just getting started or trying to add more distance. For a more advanced simulation, you can do a section of marathon pacing followed by faster interval reps to give you the feel of hard work when you are fatigued.

**Normal training run**

The basic training run should be at a comfortable length and pace. It puts time on your legs and is a moderate test you can easily recover from in 24 hours while not adding much to the deficit. You must control these as you can start to feel good, get into a rhythm, and take off, making it a much harder workout than you wanted, possibly compromising future workouts.

**Progression run**

A progression run starts at a comfortable pace and gradually goes faster to a comfortably hard pace. This could also be termed a cut-down run. You will often get faster at first as you get loose and get into a good rhythm. Then, gradually accelerate the pace. You can use distance or time segments.

**Race modeling**

This type of training takes the demands of the specific event and couples those demands into a single workout. You want to incorporate all factors, especially the end of the race. For example, if you are training for a 5000m race, you should break the race distance into segments using short breaks while simulating the paces required during various parts of the distance. You could do 5 x 1000m, the last two being faster with a 200m jog or 2 x 2000m + 2 x 500m hard, separated by 200m–400m. Think about the demands of the event and let your workout mirror those demands.

**Race pace runs**

This is like the marathon simulation. It is important so you get a feel for the specific race pace.

### Recovery run

A recovery run is like the basic training run, but it is an easier run, being relaxed and controlled. The objective is to recover from previous training, to help the body clear waste products from the muscles, and not to add to the fatigue deficit. A hard recovery run that significantly adds waste products to the muscles isn't a recovery run.

### Running with light weights

Whether running with light wrist or hand weights or running with ankle or insole weights, this should be done on a limited basis. The idea is sound: adding resistance while using good running form, challenging the specific muscles to be stronger doing the running motions. However, doing these for extended periods can lead to overuse. These weighted activities should be used more like supplements, sparingly for short periods, or as drills. Monitor these so the rhythm of movement isn't slowed.

### Sand and shallow water training

These are resistance workouts. They are great for variety and fun but are also taxing and exceedingly difficult. They can build significant strength but can also cause problems. Runners who enthusiastically jump into these, whether as a vacation variation or at a specific session, can be in an overtraining and injury mode very quickly. Recovery from a difficult workout can be longer than usual.

### Shakeout

This is a short, extremely easy run, two to five miles long. Use this to loosen up, help recovery, add miles to your training, or prepare for a workout or race later that day or the next day. It can be used as part of the race day warmup three to four hours before the race starts.

### Speed training

It is good to get speed work in twice each week. This can be an add-on or a stand-alone workout. The distance can range from 50m–200m for middle-distance runners to 800m–1600m for marathoners. Speed training can add power, coordination, and efficiency to your training. This can start at a controlled level early in the training cycle and gradually progress to your goal race. I caution you not to get carried away with your pace. Distance runners always want to show how fast they are, causing many injuries because they aren't ready to accept the demands of all-out sprinting. The speed of contraction and the range of motion required should be built over time.

**Surge training**

This is about learning how to increase the intensity for a short period in the middle of a run. Changing your rhythm isn't comfortable for most people and requires practice. The in-line single-file running workout could be an introduction to this. The group runs in a single file, and the person at the end of the line increases their pace, passing everyone to become the first person in the line. When that person gets to the front, the next person runs from the back to the front, and so on. Another way to practice would be running at a comfortably hard pace and continuously alternating speeds. Try throwing in hard sections during a distance run, as you would in a fartlek, and then go back to the pace you were running, recovering while maintaining your original pace. Or you could charge up hills while keeping a reasonable pace the rest of the time. The main idea is to insert bouts of intense running into a reasonably hard run and recover while relaxing and maintaining pace the best you can.

**Tempo run**

This controlled workout is run at a pace just below the anaerobic or lactate threshold. That pace is around the pace of a hard one-hour run or a ten-mile race, just faster than half marathon pace. If you haven't run a half marathon, take your mile pace from your last 5K, and add 20 to 30 seconds per mile for strong runners and up to 60 seconds per mile for someone just starting. I find it best to warm up and roll into

Finish a workout when you could have done one more rather than you should have done one less.

that pace I call comfortably hard. It is a controlled effort with a comfortable rhythm that isn't forced. The pace is important. Faster doesn't necessarily make this a better workout. This is designed to drive the anaerobic threshold higher, allowing you to run faster without producing excess lactates in the future. Don't make these into race efforts.

Start with a 20-minute tempo. Don't worry about distance in the beginning, as there is a learning curve on how this should feel. It takes a few tries to get comfortable. I like to have runners gradually roll into their tempo runs following their warmup because I don't want them to feel like this is a race. As you get stronger, tempos may last 40 minutes or longer. I've used straight-paced runs and progressive efforts, running the first half at pace and the second half gradually increasing to a faster but controlled run. If you start to struggle, back off the pace slightly or stop. If you want variety or to increase the time you spend at this effort, break the tempo into sections or reps, using very short recovery periods to refresh yourself.

**Time trial**

This is used to get into the race mind-set, mix in a little competition with teammates, feel the demands of the race, practice race tactics, and fill in when there are no competitions. Time trials are a great indicator of fitness. Many times, especially early in the season, I've used a distance shorter than the actual race distance.

## SUPPLEMENTAL TRAINING

Supplements to your regular training are just that, additions. Do what you should do first, then add the extras. We all must work on fitness, strength, stability, flexibility, range of motion, and balance exercises. These can aid training and help maintain fitness when injured. They aren't a substitute to prepare you for your best running.

### Buildups

Buildups are runs where you designate a distance, such as 50m, to accelerate to 70%, 80%, 90%, or 100%, and then maintain that pace for a specified distance. For instance, the overall length of the run might be 150m at 80%, indicating a 50m buildup or acceleration followed by 100m at 80% of your maximum speed. I typically incorporate these as a supplement to the workout and perform them at the end.

### Circuit training

This is a simultaneous cardio and strength workout. The idea is to work on high repetition strength while quickly going from exercise to exercise. The stations are set so that you will rotate working body parts. This requires the body to shunt blood from one muscle group to another, and so on. This gives the cardio effect. It also allows continuous activity, letting parts of the body rest while another is working. Stations can involve bodyweight exercises, medicine balls, core balls, and weights, to name a few. Examples of a 20-station circuit include bodyweight squat, back plank hamstring ball roll, push-ups on half dome, lower ab curls, Russian twists, crunches, fast up-slow down push-ups, leg flutters, squat jumps, superman lifts, bicycle twists, burpees, suitcases, mountain climbers, V-ups, jumping jacks, back plank hip raisers, front plank, side plank, continuous standing long jumps.

### Core work

Core work or pillar exercises are enormously important. The trunk of the body must be strong. When running, the legs drive the body forward.

If you push against a weak core, much of the power will dissipate, and you will lose much of the force used to move the body forward. Movements push against the main part of the body, and the body must be solid. You can find many exercises and ideas from online sources to strengthen the abs, sides, back, hips, and glutes. Mats, benches, stability balls, medicine balls, wheels, ropes, and dumbbells can enhance your ab work and planks. In addition to the regular daily core work, major core work of 30 minutes plus could be done two to three times each week. Examples include front plank, side plank, lower ab curls, Russian twists, hip flexor curl on a scooter, crunches, side crunches, leg flutters, superman lifts, bicycle twists, suitcases, mountain climbers, double-leg toss, bench jumps, V-ups, on hands and knees—opposite arm and leg, hydrants, split lunge jumps, single-leg leg raisers (toes in three positions), legs up toe touch, back plank hip raisers, and side plank lifts.

**Cross training**

These activities can significantly work your cardiovascular system while working the muscles in your body that may or may not be used in running. While these activities won't replace running, they can add to fitness without giving the same amount of pounding as running. Swimming and deep-water running can provide an intense workout, often helping to relax tight muscles. Rowing machines, stair climbers, elliptical machines, multiple kinds of arm and leg machines, rollerblading, and cycling—road, mountain, recumbent, and stationary—are all great activities. One of the best activities is cross country skiing. When I lived in Minnesota, athletes would come off their cross country skiing season with a huge engine and a strong heart. They were ready to go. And they did. One problem was that sometimes their legs weren't as prepared as their cardiovascular system to take the pounding. They needed to transition their legs back into running mode gradually, or they would run themselves into injuries.

**Finishes**

I developed a 100m to 150m three-person track drill to help runners recognize and react to what is happening in front of them. Two runners are in front and secretly decide what they'll do coming off the turn. The third runner is right behind them. The two in front can do one of three things—drift, split, or stay—Drift (both go out a lane to leave an inside opening)—Split (one stays in lane one while the other drifts out, leaving a gap between them)—or Stay (both stay inside, forcing the opening to be on the outside). I didn't allow the two runners in front to close the gap after they opened it. Although, that could be another adaptation. The purpose is to get the trailing runner to recognize what is happening in front and react to the opening. This needs to become instinctive. The runners switch positions and learn to race in the front, back, boxed in a pack, and two to three people wide. As a result, they learn to relax in all those situations.

**Flexibility**

Flexibility or stretching activities are critical. When running, you are doing the same motion over and over and over again. Muscles contract and get shorter over time with activity. You want them to be long and strong. You want a full range of motion at all joints. A long muscle is a strong muscle. You must work on maintaining a full range of motion with stretching, drills, rolling, and massage. Massage can do things that stretching can't. Restrictions can affect performance. Before the workout, after a short jog, do ballistic drills and a few selected static stretches. After the workout, do more ballistic drills, range of motion activities, and various static exercises. Pick a few exercises for each area of the body: feet, ankles, calves, quads, hamstrings, IT band, butt, hips, lower back, core, sides, arms, shoulders, and neck.

**Increase rhythm drill**

Try doing regular rhythm runs where you count the number of times your left foot hits the ground in a minute. Take a break and then try another minute to see if you can increase the number of "lefts" you can get. You would multiply this number by two to get your strides per minute.

**Magic Six**

Dr. George Sheehan passed on knowledge and philosophy about running and life. He wrote about toning the legs to help avoid injuries. His "Magic Six" helped many runners avoid missing training time due to aches and pains. He emphasized strengthening the front side of the body (crunches, quad lifts, and seated toe lifts) and stretching the back side (lying back over, standing hurdle stretch, and wall push). We can update the exercises, but the basis of this program is still solid.

**Plyometrics**

Running should be explosive with each step you take. The longer you spend on the ground, the slower you will go. Doing drills will help you develop that over time. Plyometric drills are ballistic exercises where the speed of the change of direction is as or more important than the magnitude of the jump. I've also included form, range of motion, and strength drills below to vary the stresses. Examples include heel and toe walk, bounding, light bounding, skipping, high knee skipping, little form hurdles, A-skips, B-skips, C-skips, 1000 steps, RDLs, forward and backward lunges with a medicine ball, butt kicks (two types), high knee running, backward running, fast walking, carioca, backstroke windmill, side hops with arm swings, stepping stones, straight-leg running, Frankenstein, two-legged long jumps, one and two-legged hops, squat jumps, box jumps, rope jumping, jumping jacks, and leg swings.

# Achieving a Dream

**NADINE MARKS DEMPSEY**

I met Jim Fischer while working at the University of Delaware. He asked me if I would like to be his assistant coach for the men's cross country and track & field teams. I would also be able to train with the men. I had no idea how this would change my life.

While helping to coach the men, I was training harder than I had my entire life. I remember the weekly training regimen that consisted of a long run, track or hill workout, tempo run, speed work, and easy days in between. My favorite run was the 8 a.m. Sunday morning long run. We would run anywhere from ten to 15 miles. Monday would be an easy five-mile run followed by a hard mile on the track.

I must admit, I did not like doing that at all. On Tuesday, we would do either a track workout or hill workout. These would be intense, and I would be exhausted afterward. The 6 a.m. Thursday morning tempo run was tough, but I felt so accomplished when I was finished. We would run out and back on Creek Road, and the goal was to negative split. I usually did three miles, but the men would sometimes do as many as five or six miles. Coming back in the afternoon, we would be on the track for 200-meter repeats. I loved the feeling of running fast. Saturday would be race day and time to put all that hard work to use. I remember some races where I felt like I was floating. I was running so fast, and yet it felt so effortless. My coach had prepared me well!

In 2000, I was sponsored by Saucony. To my amazement, I was running somewhat professionally! Coach Fischer gave so much of his time to help me succeed and achieve my running goals. I set PRs for everything from 800m to the half marathon. I was in the best shape of my life and had hopes of making it to the Olympic Trials.

In 2002, I represented the USA at the Beijing Ekiden. I was so excited to be competing internationally. I was running great, and my dreams continued until I suffered a career-ending injury. Unfortunately, this would be my last race. I had stopped competing at a time when I was consistently improving. I regret not knowing just how good I could have been and if I would have made it to the Olympic Trials, but I look back on that time with a feeling of accomplishment as well. I never would have had any of those opportunities had it not been for Coach Fischer.

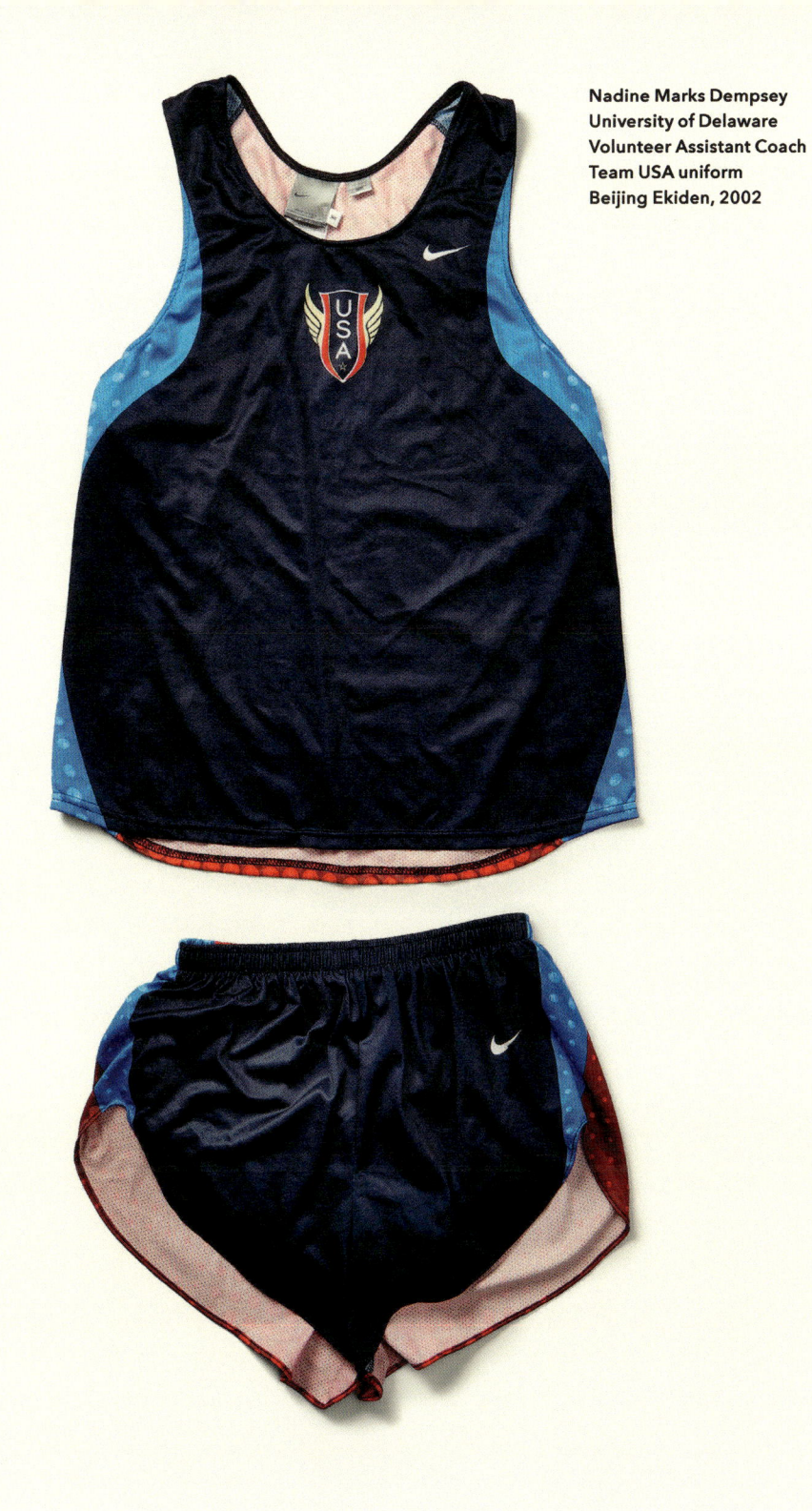

Nadine Marks Dempsey
University of Delaware
Volunteer Assistant Coach
Team USA uniform
Beijing Ekiden, 2002

RUN. **TRAIN.** RACE.

## Pool training

Pool training can be a great workout. You can use a belt or go without it (which usually turns out to be a tougher workout). You can do regular swimming strokes or deep-water activities such as running and strength work. An injured athlete can even do the same workout the rest of the team does, only in deep water. It is highly effective in rehabilitation as you can get your heart rate elevated by working against the strong resistance of the water but not have the pounding. I've found that even short sessions in the pool, while very fatiguing, work to relieve tightness and let the muscles relax afterward. This can be great for recovery. Invariably, people feel much better the day after a water workout.

## Strength work

Strength activities are essential, whether it is weight training, bodyweight exercises, or functional training, and should cover weaknesses, maximize strengths, and correct imbalances. It can be doing a bodyweight circuit, using bands, pushing a sled, or spending time in the weight room. The body needs to be strong from head to toe. Bulky muscles are always an issue or fear. This shouldn't be a problem. Using lighter weights, higher repetitions, and a full range of motion are things to remember when building basic strength or maintaining strength during the competitive season. Distance runners focus on their legs in running workouts, and many don't want to "lift" with their legs. I've found that lifting with your legs is especially important. There is a compelling case for having heavier, lower-rep leg work during the off- and early-season training. Many leg exercises would enhance running and add balance to the body, helping to ward off injuries. Core and hip strength are essential. The body's trunk provides a stable pillar around which the running action occurs. You want your whole body toned.

You want to balance your strength front and back, side to side, upper and lower body. This doesn't mean that opposing muscles will be equal in strength. It does mean that deficits can cause a pulling of one body part in a slightly different direction than where it was supposed to be pulled. For example, quad strength to hamstring strength should be about three to two. In distance runners, the quads are usually weaker. This can cause strains or patellar tracking problems. At a minimum, you could gain muscle tone by doing straight-leg leg raisers, one leg at a time, ten with the toes pointed out, ten with the toes pointed up, and ten with the toes pointed in. You won't gain much strength, but increased muscle tone might solve the problem.

The upper body must be strong as well. The arms are a dynamic part of running. Weaknesses here show up in performances. Think of holding your arms in the same relative position, doing the same motion over and over for hours in a marathon. The day after my first marathon, I thought someone had pulled my arms out of their sockets. Think of the dynamics of movement in the final moments of a 5K. Those take strength. Also, weaknesses could mean that your body mechanics could be moving inefficiently. It sounds like a contradiction, but upper body strength is essential for relaxation in addition to being able to hold proper form. Examples of weight room exercises include tricep dips, lat pulls, side lifts with weight, back plank hamstring ball roll, lying weighted hip thrusts, lower ab ball curls, upright rows, seated row, single-leg RDL, perfect plank push-ups, sit-ups holding weight, overhead press, bench press, arm curls. In addition, functional training equipment such as strength bands, tubing, stability balls, balance stability pieces, medicine balls, TRX trainers, exercise wheels, ropes, kettlebells, plyo boxes, and many more can add so much to training.

**Striders**

These are fast, relaxed runs, usually 50m to 100m long, and paced halfway between a jog and a sprint. The emphasis is on good, relaxed form with solid turnover and rhythm. Imagine that you are being filmed and you want to look good. They can be incorporated into the warmup and warm-down. These can also be done barefoot on smooth grass to strengthen the lower legs and feet small muscles, tendons, and ligaments.

## 10s and body weight 10s

These are groups of ten activities that combine lightweight and bodyweight exercises like hopping, throwing, lifting, and strengthening that can be done at the end of a workout. They can be used when no formal weight training equipment is available or as a supplement to the strength training program. These are for gradual strengthening over the long term. Examples include 10s—toe raisers/calf stretch, balance pods, bands, light shoulder weights, box jumps, forward and backward lunges/medicine ball, hurdle hops, rope jump, kettlebell goblet squats, kneeling hamstring curls, 10s BW—body weight squats, fast up-slow down push-ups, lower ab curls, 3-step side shuffle, six-count burpees, slow Russian twists, back plank hip raisers, mountain climbers, standing long jumps, a variety of front planks.

## Single-leg strength and balance drills (S.L. series)

Physical therapist Andrew "Rudy" Rudawsky gave me a series of single-leg strength and balance drills that are great for runners. Do ten to 30 reps of each exercise on one leg and then the other non-stop. They are running woman (or man), open the gate, close the gate, squat with opposite leg forward, squat with opposite leg to the side, squat with the opposite leg backward. Hold the following on one leg and then the other non-stop for ten to 30 seconds each: knee to chest, knee to the opposite shoulder, knee to the outside, hip hike, piriformis stretch, quad stretch, and RDL.

## Warmup, form, and strength drills

You must always warm up for your cold muscles to work properly. But, if you go to the other extreme, overheating, your performance will also be impaired as you work harder and the core temperature increases. The warmup should enhance, not hurt, performance, no matter how long it is. Without a proper warmup, your maximum heart rate can be ten to 20 beats per minute lower than following a full warmup. I can't tell you the number of times I've heard people say they didn't get rolling and warmed up until halfway through the race. If running a long-distance race, do an "efficient" warmup to prepare yourself. It is OK to use the first mile or two to get into your rhythm if you are new to the distance, if your training is limited, or if you are unsure of your training. For a shorter distance race, it shouldn't negatively impact performance if you feel you need to do a two- or three-mile warmup to ensure you are ready to go when the gun goes off. If it does, you need to get into better shape!

These dynamic drills can strengthen the body, reinforce good running mechanics, and provide solid preparation for workouts and races.

## DYNAMIC DRILLS

| | |
|---|---|
| **Heel and toe walk** | Walk first on your heels without toes touching the ground, then walk on tiptoes with heels not touching the ground |
| **Light bounding, bounding** | Exaggerated running with emphasis on covering as much distance as possible with every step, keeping the upper body upright and relaxed, and spending as little time on the ground as possible—light or strong |
| **Diagonal bounding (stepping stones)** | Same as above, except make each step at a 45° angle |
| **Carioca** | Sideways "grapevine" running with strong rotation of the opposite leg leading in front of the body with each step, bringing the knee up, and returning in the other direction with the other leg leading in front of the body |
| **High knee running** | Quick running with high knee action |
| **Skipping, high knee skipping** | Childhood skipping—normal or explosive to gain both height and distance with each step |

| | |
|---|---|
| **Little form hurdles** | Running over hurdles while maintaining posture, form, and rhythm with lifted knees |
| **RDLs** | Take a couple steps and then bend at waist with a straight back (no arch) to lift one leg straight back—alternate legs |
| **Forward and backward lunges** | Walking, alternating single-leg forward to thigh parallel to the ground with alignment of knees directly above feet (not extending past toes)—can add medicine ball |
| **1000 steps** | Fast steps with toes hitting the ground as quickly as possible |
| **Frankenstein** | Straight-leg walking, high toe touch without bending knees |
| **Straight leg running (drum major)** | Quickly moving with straight body leaning slightly backwards, and moving arms fast in running motion |
| **Butt kicks (two types)** | A slow run in which the heels bend backwards to touch butt, with knees pointed down or high knees |
| **Single- and two-legged hops** | Jumping forward, trying to cover as much distance as possible |
| **Two-legged long jumps** | Jumping simultaneously with both legs, trying to cover as much distance as possible |
| **Backstroke windmill** | Walking with opposite arm sweeping high overhead |
| **Fast walking** | Walking fast emphasizing arm swing and toe push-off |
| **Side hops with arm swings (lateral jumping jacks)** | Sideways hopping, alternating arms meeting above the head and below the waist |

| | |
|---|---|
| **Box jumps** | Jumping up and down off a box as quickly as possible |
| **Squat jumps** | Squat with feet shoulder width apart, a straight back with knees bent, then jump as high as possible, landing and into another jump as quickly as possible |
| **Rope jumping** | Single- and two-legged rope jumping for quickness and duration |
| **Backward running** | Running backward with tall posture |
| **Leg swings** | Swinging one leg at a time in large sweeping motions, rotating from the hip |
| **A-skips** | Good form skipping |
| **B-skips** | Good form skipping with an added extension of the leg in a pawing motion once reaching the highest point of skip |
| **C-skips** | Alternate skipping—bouncing on toes, only one knee at a time raise, beginning with right knee (and toe) pointed to the side touches ground then quickly raises up, right toe touches ground then rotates to be forward with high knee and then touches ground, then left knee raises up in forward direction and touches ground, then left knee rotates to side and touches ground, left knee then raises up, continue back to left leg forward, and then back to right leg forward, then right leg side, and so on |

If you have a weakness, the race will find it.

## PUTTING IT TOGETHER—PERIODIZATION

If you have a weakness, the race will find it. It doesn't matter how good you are or your motivation; many things will be revealed when you finish. Some of the things might be good, and some not so much. The race will indicate where you are with your conditioning, strategy, and competitiveness.

The planning process is called periodization in track & field and distance running. While we want the ability to be flexible, there needs to be a plan or training cycle on how to fit everything into the schedule. Having all the perfect ingredients doesn't mean success. This all must be put together correctly. Some objectives regarding endurance, speed, coordination, and psychological aspects related to your goals are to be developed. You can plan your progression of volume or miles and the amount of intensity work to be done. You can schedule when you will race and determine the importance of each race.

This plan should include what you want to work on and when. You start with a broad outline and gradually get more and more specific. The whole cycle can be divided into five phases. First, there needs to be time to develop basic fitness, focusing on your cardiovascular base or foundation and doing some basic intensity work to break the monotony and keep you in touch with your leg speed. Second, you need time to develop specific fitness, build strength, and learn to tolerate and recover from hard work. This work is added to the foundation you built during the first phase. As you go through this phase, workouts should gradually increase in specificity. The closer the training focuses on the things needed to be successful, the SAID Principle (Specific Adaptation to Imposed Demand), the better the results. Third, there is a learning and developmental phase when you work on racing intensity, tactics, and techniques. Fourth, this is the phase when you want all your work to culminate in being able to compete to the full extent of your potential. Lastly, there needs to be a phase to mend and heal physically, mentally, and emotionally, rest and rebuild, and freshen before the next cycle starts the process all over again at a higher level. You build volume first, add strength work, and the volume drops as the intensity increases. This cycle or some variation may last four months, six months, nine months, twelve months, or however long you choose.

Many in the public sector will use a twelve-month cycle, using the winter months for their transition or resting period and endurance-building time. Coaches use various cycles in a school setting, depending on where and when they want their emphasis to be. The athletes would go through their endurance, strength, competition, and resting periods to become stronger each training cycle. If, at the end of their cycle, they were at the same level as when they arrived, either their perceived effort should be lower, or something went wrong. Most of the time, I use two six-month cycles per year, one starting on June 1st and another on December 1st, with cross country and outdoor track & field being the main focal seasons.

Some will disagree with me on this next point, but that's okay. Back in college, when I was still a math major, I worked hard and spent almost all my time on the most challenging courses, and the grades I received were a few B's and some C's. With all the effort I put into those courses, I had limited time to spend on the easy ones and also got B's and some C's. That wasn't working for me. So, I switched. I went after getting good grades in my easy courses and still spent a reasonable amount of time on the challenging courses, just not almost all my time. This brought me to a philosophy I've transferred to other things: maximizing my strengths and covering my weaknesses. Do the things you do well very well. Cover the things you don't do well as best you can. Working tirelessly on things you don't do well will waste valuable time and energy and may compromise the things you do well.

It is a good idea for you to think several years into the future. As you move from one cycle to the next and the next and so on, some aspects must get stronger each time. You might want your weekly mileage to be higher so that you do a larger volume of intensity during each workout. Alternatively, your goal could be to have your hard workouts at a higher level of intensity. Perhaps, you want to maintain the same level of everything but concentrate on having your perceived effort be lower for the same level of training. If you are working to improve and are still at the same level of performance years later, either you are old enough to try to cover what Father Time is taking from you, or you need to adjust something in your training as you aren't improving.

Some coaches have a training philosophy that uses a low mileage with a high-intensity approach, while others prefer high mileage with moderately high intensity. Most are somewhere in between, doing a moderate amount of weekly mileage and hard workouts to test the athletes but limiting the very high-intensity workouts. Some train using distance for measuring their workouts, some use time, and some use a combination of both. Many go with their comfort level and what works for them.

The total volume of distance or time each week should be monitored. If you do a two-mile, a five-mile, or a 45-minute run, depending on how you track it, write it down in a log, sum a total for a week, and view the stability or progression of your overall training. Likewise, note the total volume of the meters or minutes of intensity on any day you do a hard workout. If you do six times 800m, the total of 4800m should be charted for that day. Warmup, warm-down, and recovery running would be counted in the total daily volume but not in the daily intensity volume. Considering that your training goal is similar from week to week, you shouldn't have huge increases in that total. Increases in the weekly amount of running volume and the daily total amount of intensity should be gradual. During the training cycle, taking a "down" week every three to four weeks is good. That would mean you would decrease the amount you ran and the total intensity for that week to aid your overall recovery. The level of intensity would stay the same unless you need extra recovery.

## TRAINING STRUCTURE

My daily schedule emphasizes a gradually stronger dynamic warmup, increasing in intensity to prepare the body for the workout, and a gradually relaxing, calming warm-down after the workout, decreasing in intensity to bring the body back to normal. It is like a pyramid. Use this general model for your daily workouts: short, slow warmup jog to get the blood flowing into the muscles, dynamic form, rotation, preparation, and range of motion drills, light stretching, warmup run, light stretching, striders on the day of intensity workouts, the main workout that you have planned, warm-down run, striders, stretching, strength drills, dynamic and static stretching, core work, strength work, and an optional short shake-out run.

The time of the warmup should approximately equal the time of the warm-down. The objectives are to prepare for activity by gradually raising the body temperature and loosening the muscles, doing the workout, and, after, gradually decreasing the intensity to lower the body temperature. The warmup at the beginning makes the muscles, tendons, and ligaments more pliable and promotes a full range of motion. The warm-down at the end lets you stretch muscles, tendons, and ligaments that are pliable, helps to clear waste products, and promotes nutrient distribution to the cells to begin the healing process. You want a great range of motion in your whole body. Don't stretch to the point of pain, ever!

On resistance training days, whether the training is bodyweight, free weights, machines, balls, bands, ropes, etc., do a majority of the running part of the training first so you can concentrate on control during the workout. Sometimes, you could do strength work before the workout to imitate extreme fatigue, with the idea that you would want to learn to stay relaxed and under control even when tired. Hand, insole, and ankle weights during a running workout could be used on a limited basis for gaining strength. If you use them regularly for a whole workout, they may cause your normal running rhythm to slow and lead to overuse injuries.

## THIS IS A BASIC STRUCTURE OF A DAILY WORKOUT

1. Short, slow warmup jog
2. Dynamic drills—form, plyometric, strength, and range of motion
3. Light stretching—a few easy stretches, especially on trouble spots
4. Warmup run—easy run for a minimum of 10 minutes
5. Light stretching—a few easy stretches on places that still feel tight
6. Striders—4 to 8 x 50m-100m
7. Main workout
8. Warm-down run—easy relaxed run for a minimum of 10 minutes
9. Striders—4 to 8 x 50mm-100m
10. Stretching—concentrated overall body stretching
11. Strength drills
12. Dynamic & static stretching
13. Core work
14. Strength work
15. Easy jog

Think of all the repetitions in a single 30-minute run, let alone doing it every day. However, most of the time, you want to do strength work at the end of the workout, so there would be no question as to whether or not you could control all aspects of the running for that day. Try this. Write your name, do 20 push-ups, then write your name again. How much control did you have the second time you wrote your name?

### FOUR-DAY TRAINING SCHEDULE

|  | Sunday | Monday | Tuesday |
|---|---|---|---|
| **OPTION 1** | Long run | Off | Easy run |
| **OPTION 2** | Easy run | Off | Interval workout |
| **OPTION 3** | Long run | Easy run | Off |

### SIX- OR SEVEN-DAY TRAINING SCHEDULE

|  | Sunday | Monday | Tuesday |
|---|---|---|---|
| **OPTION 1** | Long run | Easy run | Interval workout |
| **OPTION 2** | Long run | Easy run | Interval workout |
| **OPTION 3** | Easy run or off | Interval workout | Easy run |

Let me give you a few weekly training schedule options. The number of possibilities is endless. These will give you an idea of what I mean.

The basic schedule is hard-easy, hard one day and easy the next. Interval workouts and tempo runs can be done on a track, trail, grass, or road. Days can be shifted. Supplemental activities can be added.

| Wednesday | Thursday | Friday | Saturday |
| --- | --- | --- | --- |
| Off | Tempo run | Off | Easy run |
| Off | Easy run | Off | Long run |
| Tempo run | Off | Easy run | Off |

| Wednesday | Thursday | Friday | Saturday |
| --- | --- | --- | --- |
| Easy run or off | Tempo run | Easy run | Fartlek or easy run |
| Easy run or off | Easy run | Tempo run | Easy run |
| Easy run | Tempo run | Easy run | Long run |

Below are more specific mileage examples of training schedules. I'm not listing the particular workouts, just approximate daily distances for corresponding weekly mileages. These are only sample schedules and can be altered to fit each person's needs.

| MILES/WEEK | 25 | 45 | 65 | 85 | 105 | 125 |
|---|---|---|---|---|---|---|
| Sunday | 8 | 10 | 13 | 17 | 20 | 23 |
| Monday | Off | 6 | 8 | 10 | 12 | 16 |
| Tuesday | 6 | 8 | 10 | 15 | 18 | 18 |
| Wednesday | Off | Off | 8 | 10 | 12 | 16 |
| Thursday | 6 | 8 | 10 | 15 | 18 | 18 |
| Friday | Off | 7 | 8 | 8 | 12 | 16 |
| Saturday | 5 | 6 | 8 | 10 | 13 | 18 |

To those working with athletes in high school or college, I scheduled weekend workouts in the morning to help them realize that it would be a good idea to get to bed early so they get enough sleep the night before a workout.

When you are training five, six, or seven days per week, your workout week should have a long day (longest and slowest day of the week), a hard day (hills, intervals, fartlek, etc.), and a tempo day. Another intensity day (a race or an especially hilly run) can be added, but recovery is vital. Three days of hard workouts or races plus a long run can be a tough week. More work isn't always better.

Fixed training schedules that you find in books and magazines are good. The schedule shows you a structure that is needed. There are usually schedules for beginners, intermediates, and advanced athletes. They get you going in the right direction. However, some people have a compulsive adherence to a generic schedule. They look at a schedule and say that they must do this workout on this day, and if they don't, it will mess up their training, and their race performance will suffer. People aren't all the same.

I was one of those people. I had a 20-mile run scheduled. It snowed 20 inches. I still went out and did it because it was on the schedule. It was a lot of work, and I was tired when I finished. I was tired days later. It affected my training for at least a week. Then I realized that I could have done it another day, shortened it, or not done it at all. I know that runners want to be consistent. You need to learn that, but you have to get all your training elements in the correct order. If you have trouble getting out the door to run, you need that schedule staring you in the face. You need that schedule for guidance. I get it! After you've learned to be consistent, you must learn how to adjust. Life, facility availability, weather, schedules, work, relationships, time, energy, and fatigue get in the way. What are the essential things you need to do, and what compromises or adaptations can be made so you can still be successful?

Many highly competitive athletes run twice a day for most of the week. One of the workouts is usually shorter and less intense. With everything you must cover, more elements of your training program can be included in the additional workouts. It is easier to run more miles daily and to maintain a higher quality of work by splitting it into two sessions. This also means that you must get out the door twice. This is generally for the highly competitive runner who can determine this individually.

If you're struggling, you can stop the workout any time. You aren't in the middle of the ocean.

An example of a general workout schedule for someone competing at a high level might use these principles. They might push things to another day or in a different sequence. Athletes will do a second shorter workout on many of these days.

## DAYS AND WORKOUTS

| | | |
|---|---|---|
| **Sunday** | Long run | Slowest day of the week |
| **Monday** | Recovery/Prep | Average workout length, recovery from previous training and racing, prep for the next day with a small amount of controlled intensity |
| **Tuesday** | Hard workout | A major workout of the week |
| **Wednesday** | Recovery | Easy day to recover from Tuesday |
| **Thursday** | Tempo/Turnover work | 2-10 miles, depending on racing distance, at roughly the pace you could run for 10 miles, controlled, not raced, take a break or later in the day, do 2000m-3000m of short runs of 200m, 300m, or 400m to add turnover training |
| **Friday** | Recovery/Prep | Shorter than average workout length, recovery from previous training, prep for race or workout the next day with a small amount of controlled intensity |
| **Saturday** | Flexible day | Race, Fartlek, Hills, Hard workout, Long day, Recovery day, or Zero day |

## DOING WORKOUTS

Train to run another day. Workouts are the vehicle to reach the destination, not the final destination. You can feel excited about completing a workout and what it means for your training and confidence, but that's as far as it should go. The main goal is competition. The goal of the training should be maximal-specific fitness for the performances you want. Gradually let your training make the adaptations. Strenuous workouts, whether from high intensity, high mileage, or just plain work, need to be followed by enough recovery time to strengthen the body. If you can't recover from a hard workout in 24–48 hours, you may have done too much unless that's what you wanted. Most times, if you are wiped out, you may have done yourself a disservice as you have compromised your training schedule and may need extra days to recover. My friend, Art Gulden, who coached at Bucknell University, often said, "Don't write checks that your body can't cash."

There are some non-negotiables. If you want to get better at running, you must run. You can cross-train by doing other activities, and in many cases, it will help to balance your opposing muscles, fill deficits, help rehabilitate or avoid injuries, and give variety to your life. Cross-training can help you to maintain and elevate your cardiovascular fitness and muscle strength but is limited in what it will do for your performance. Training is specific. You need to run. Taking that further, if you want to run fast, you will eventually have to train fast.

In distance running, strength is speed. For me, the central part of this is cardiovascular strength. You can reach much of your potential by getting in good shape. Running fast repetitions will help the efficiency of movement, intensify strength, and get you to your maximum potential. You can and should be doing fast reps during most of your training cycle. However, most of your "speed" will come from doing regular training, teaching the body to recover more quickly through day after day running, completing hill repeats and hilly trails, flowing through fartlek and interval workouts, cruising through tempos, persevering through long runs, doing core work, body weight exercises, flexibility, and weight training. You can't rely on fast stuff alone to get where you want to go. You must do all the work.

Workouts are measured on their duration (minutes, miles, or kilometers), the amount of intensity work (minutes or meters), and the density (the ratio of the repetition length to the amount of recovery). These are all manipulated depending on the point the athlete is at in their training.

Generally, once the repetition length is determined, the number of reps is set by the desired number of meters of intensity. The speed of the rep will vary depending on the point in the training cycle. The average recovery is usually half the distance or equal to the rep's time. That can change depending on the objectives of the workout. The rest might be longer for high-intensity workouts, and lower-intensity workouts have shorter rest periods. Most of the time, recovery periods will involve jogging. Again, the manipulation of five variables—the length of the repetition (time or distance), the number of repetitions, the speed of repetitions, the length of recovery (time or distance), and the nature of recovery (slower run, jog, walk, stand, etc.)—will rely on the desired effect of the workout.

For general training, interval repetitions of 400m and 600m reps are run at sub 3K pace, 800m to 1200m reps at 5K pace, and 1600m to 2400m reps in the 10K range. As the athlete becomes more experienced and moves to a more intense training program, the pace ranges increase with the 400m, and 600m reps run closer to goal 3K pace and then on to mile pace, the 800m to 1200m reps to goal 5K and on to 3K pace, and the 1600m to 2400m reps to goal 10K pace and on to 5K pace. These approximations will change depending on the workout's goal and the place in the training progression.

I want the second half of every workout to be as fast as or faster than the first half. Every workout is at least partly a progressive workout. This doesn't mean that every workout should hammer you into submission. Many people tell me they slowed down during the second half of their workout. They tell me they felt so good during the first half but so bad during the second half and slowed dramatically. That's because they didn't pace properly. Make sure you are warmed up. Resist the temptation to go too fast during the first half of the workout. You may need to artificially start slowly or at least not run faster than you are supposed to run. The workout should increase in intensity as it progresses. It is about control and getting to know the feeling of what you can handle and what you can't. It is also about practicing being strong physically, mentally, and emotionally at the end, whether it is a workout or a race.

While doing a workout, especially where you are doing repetitions, whether on a track, at a park, or wherever, make sure that you run through to the end. Many times, in races, people run a great race, only to ease up five to ten meters before the finish line and someone passes them. For some, this has little importance. For others, this may mean an age group placing, a medal, prize money, a race win, or a berth on the Olympic Team. They couldn't wait to slow down when they only had to go a little further. They didn't save that much energy. They just wanted the pain to be over. This mistake can be corrected by never slowing down before the finish line or the end of a repetition in any workout. Get in the habit of running all the way to the end, or as my coaching mentor, Roy Griak, said, ten meters past the finish line.

Train smart, not simply hard. A workout will have the purpose of working on specific objectives. Run the pace that will meet the planned objectives. But training smart also includes knowing when to finish a workout early for various reasons. A good rule of thumb is to stop a workout when you feel you could do one more rep rather than when you should have done one less. It should be before you are already extremely fatigued or have started to struggle. Remember that you are in control and can stop at any time. Don't keep going just to finish the workout; it will lead to longer recovery and potential injuries. Sure, there are times when you might want to test yourself and go to near exhaustion, a "gut check," if you will. Those times should be few, and you should ensure that you fully recover before you do another intense workout.

Stopping a workout may take just as much mental toughness as finishing it. A "hungry" athlete who wants to work, wants to improve, wants to fight the pain, and doesn't look for ways to get out of work will have the confidence that they'll be stronger next time. For some athletes, stopping a workout may lead to a vicious cycle where they are hesitant to start the next workout for fear that they won't be able to complete it or meet expectations. Or they may not want to get into the habit of stopping whenever they start to feel uncomfortable. Regardless of the reason for stopping early, the trust between a coach and an athlete, as well as within the athletes themselves, will be tested. If an athlete stops because they want to get out of doing the work, that's on them. But, if they are truly done and can't effectively do anymore, they need to stop.

I'm always disappointed when a workout can't be completed. I'm not disappointed with the person; I'm disappointed for them. I trust that they want to get better even more than I want them to. I trust that they won't try to skip or avoid a workout. But that trust, like many things, must be developed and earned. I've had runners think of every excuse to get out of workouts, especially athletes just starting. People who are deeply committed to reaching their potential will do everything possible to complete all the work. Then, when I see them struggling, or they come and tell me that they can't do any more work, there is no question that the next step is warming down and coming back to train another day. There is no workout so important that it had to be done that day. That is why consistency of training minimizes the effect of a missed or shortened workout.

Noel Relyea
Western States
Endurance Run
Award, 1991

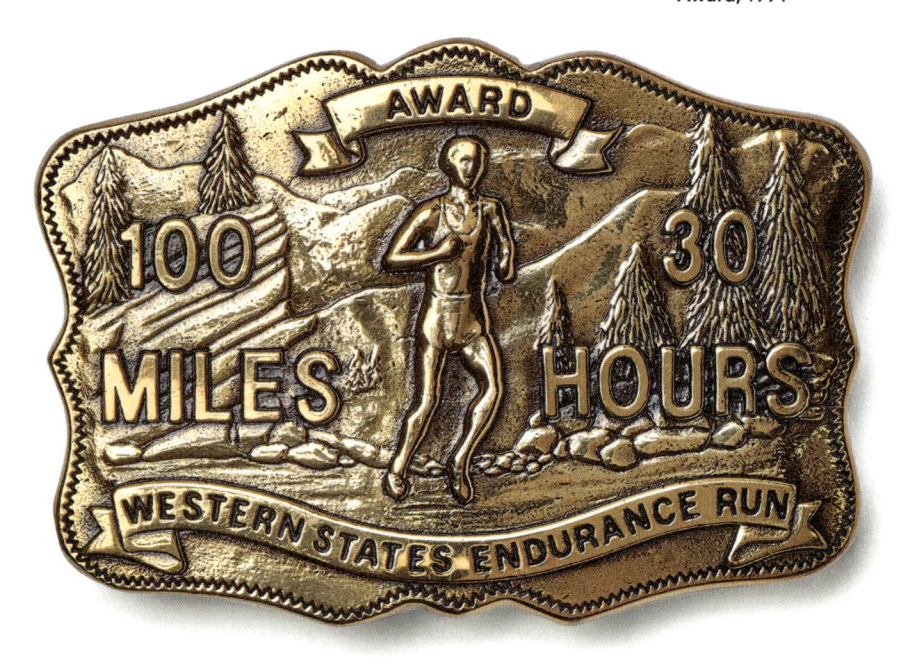

# My First 100-miler

**NOEL RELYEA**

It's amazing to me how much difference a pacer can make in a race. Pacers are allowed in most ultras so that runners don't get lost in the darkness during the final nighttime stretch. Running in an ultramarathon is as much mental as it is physical. It's critical to know that you can do it. When I ran my first 100-miler, the Western States 100, Jim Fischer agreed to be my pacer for the final 20 miles. It may well have been a low point in his impressive career when he was relegated to luring me ahead with the promise of bits of a Snickers bar during the final miles. But it was definitely a high point for me to manage to finish my first 100-miler.

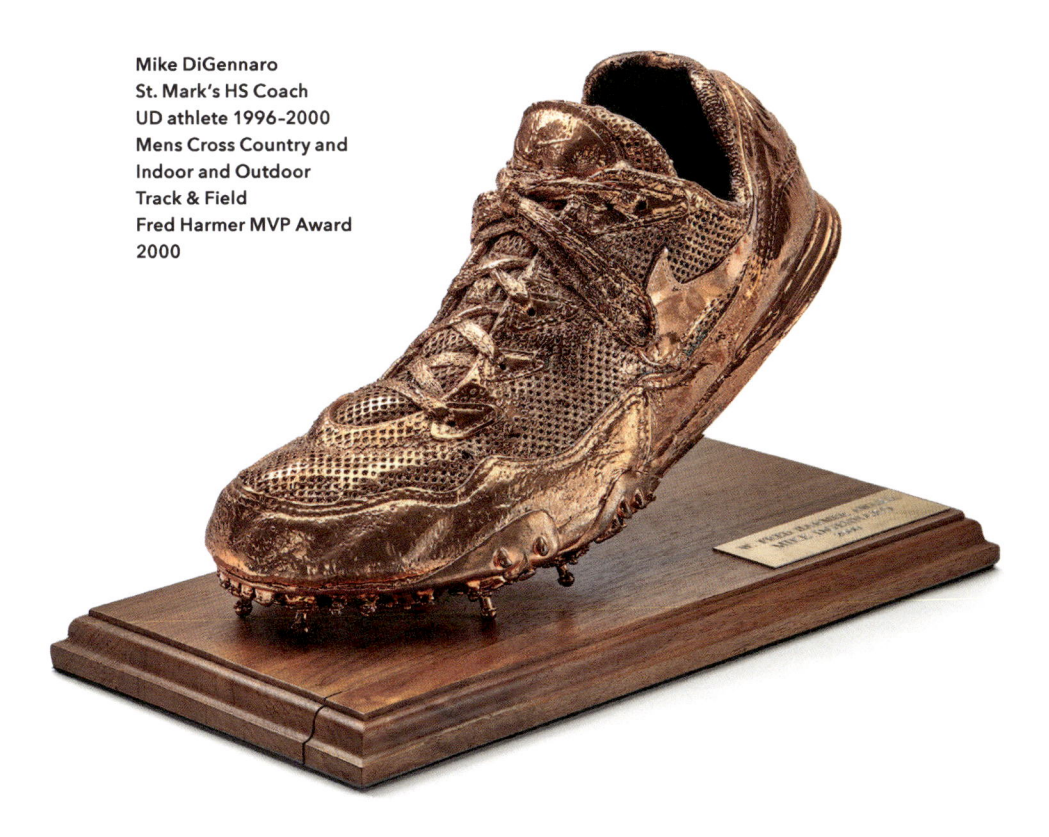

Mike DiGennaro
St. Mark's HS Coach
UD athlete 1996-2000
Mens Cross Country and
Indoor and Outdoor
Track & Field
Fred Harmer MVP Award
2000

# Bronzed Shoe

**MIKE DIGENNARO**

My college cross country journey began as a redshirt freshman, where I finished last in a race of over 150 runners at Van Cortlandt Park, covering 8K in 29:30. Four years later, in my fifth-year senior season at the IC4A Championship at the same venue, I seized the lead with 600 meters to go and won my final race as a Blue Hen in 24:50. Van Cortlandt Park marked the starting point and culmination of my growth from an inexperienced runner to a confident veteran.

The bronzed shoe, my 1998 Nike Eldoret track spike, was worn in all my senior races at UD and retired as the MVP award for the outdoor track & field team. This award is particularly meaningful as our team won the American East Conference Championship, and it was determined by a team vote, making it a memorable year as a Blue Hen.

Managing fatigue is critical. Fatigue can be cumulative, building over time. The term "burned out" is often an excuse meaning recovery that wasn't managed very well. If you are getting weaker instead of stronger, you are doing something wrong. Rest and recovery are equal partners with the work you do. Learn the difference between good tired and bad tired, good hurt and bad hurt. I use a car analogy that helps me think about fatigue and what the ramifications are. A car has a frame that's built extraordinarily strong to protect us. As the car gets higher and higher mileage, the shocks and the springs wear out. The weaker they become, the higher the stress on the frame. Taken to an extreme, some parts of the frame could fail, resulting in structural damage. The human body has a frame, the skeleton, made up of many bones. The muscles, ligaments, and tendons are the shocks and springs of the body, propelling us and protecting us from stresses caused by movements, jarring, and jolts. As the muscles, ligaments, and tendons get fatigued, the skeleton takes more and more abuse until some part fails. It is a gradual and constant process to strengthen the muscles, tendons, and ligaments to handle anything we impose on them. Training teaches the body to adapt to stress. Through it all, it is important to maintain a positive attitude. With so many aches and pains, good days and bad days, you must understand that you need to do the things that will change the bad days into good days.

Two workouts in a day, or doubles, challenge the body to recover more quickly. When trying this for the first time, it would be best to do it once or twice weekly and then continue a limited schedule. Your body will get used to this schedule but initially balk at this extra abuse. It is an effective way to increase your mileage slowly. If you are wondering whether to split your daily mileage, there are several variables to consider. Is a four-mile run in the morning and a six-mile run at night worth the same as doing a ten-mile run all at once? A ten-mile run done all at once is more challenging than splitting the distance into four and six miles. Splitting it won't stress you as much, but you must get out the door twice.

Doing the mileage all at once would be a stronger training stimulus. However, it might be too much if you are struggling with fatigue. You must ask yourself some questions. Will a ten-mile run cause me to take an extra day to recover or injure me? Will splitting the mileage help me do more training and strengthen me faster? Do I need the stress of one sustained run to get used to that challenge? Is it harder to get out the door twice on the same day? Do I only have one time during the day that I can run? There are other questions, but you get the picture. Make decisions on what you can handle and your future goals.

The last major workout is about eight to ten days before THE RACE. After recovering from that workout, do maintenance work. This should include some fast-paced but shorter workouts to stay in touch with your turnover and speed but relaxed at a decreased total volume. You can't do much to help yourself in those last few days, but you can do things that can hurt. Prepare to run well.

Get used to the pain involved with training; get comfortable with being uncomfortable. It can be uncomfortable for most when just starting. Just going out for a run isn't always the nirvana we are all looking for, as no matter how slow you go, some work is involved. We all need to develop a sense of mental toughness. But then, if you decide to take that next step into training and possibly to racing, there will be times when you will be uncomfortable and maybe even in pain, the good kind. Some embrace the pain or even look forward to it. Pain indicates that you are working to improve, but pain can also mean you are doing too much. You must be able to learn to tell the difference.

Training for improvement can be like walking along the edge of a cliff. You are trying to push yourself to your limits while working to keep from falling over the edge. With training, it is a risk/reward situation. You want to train hard to become better. You may even want to explore your limits. Critical points of diminishing returns vary from person to person regarding your work. Those points are the difference between getting stronger or risking injury and illness. Setbacks, injuries, and illnesses are part of the game. Elite athletes aren't immune. With gained awareness, you can limit the downtime you will experience.

When should you work out? The answers are too numerous to mention. Life gets in the way. Work out when you can—morning, noon, or night. Working out in the early morning means you aren't warmed up and must start more slowly, in addition to the possible lack of sleep. Trying to squeeze in a workout at noon usually means you have something to do at either end of the workout in addition to showering, which will shorten the time or make the experience uncomfortable or rushed. Doing an evening workout may mean fitting it in around meals and family activities, in addition to dealing with a layer of fatigue from your busy day. Things to consider include work or school times, meetings, the schedules of training partners, transportation, time, the kids' drop-off/pick-up times, convenience, events, track or course availability, social calendar, daylight, meals, family schedules, and so on. It would be best to have a consistent schedule, but it isn't always possible. Do the best you can and keep your stress and anxiety levels under control.

## USING YOUR WATCH

There is an ongoing discussion regarding whether one should wear a watch. Many people want to know how far they have gone based on either time or distance. Most experienced runners are very well attuned to their approximate pace because they have often run specific paces. They can determine their distance by how long they have been running. Others have mileposts or mile markers on their routes so they can evaluate their pace. During track workouts, the watch will give you immediate feedback on your running pace. For some, this clock-watching becomes obsessive and can take the fun out of training. Now, watches give us so much information that we can obsess too much about distance and pace. Some finish a training run and run around a parking lot for 17 seconds to end their run at an even number. If they are too fast in a race or workout, they fret they won't be able to finish or will feel pain for a long time. If they are too slow, they worry about what is wrong, will miss their goal, and will struggle to make up the time.

Learning to have a "feel" for your pace is extremely important. It can be so freeing not to be constrained by a watch. You should also learn how your body functions on that day and at that time—perceived effort. Get into a rhythm, and don't struggle with your pace. If you struggle, try to work your way into a good rhythm. Sometimes, you must discard the watch and listen to your body. This is especially true when you are tired, recovering from a hard workout or race, or the weather is awful. The main danger in discarding your watch is that you might get going too fast without it, possibly postponing your recovery.

A specific place where feel will come in handy is during workouts. If you plan to do a workout at 5K pace and there is a brutal wind that you will have to contend with, you should run the workout at 5K effort. Your times may be slower, but you are still making the effort. Suppose you attempt to run your 5K pace. In that case, you will probably be working much harder than usual, making it a tougher workout than you wanted or expected requiring a longer recovery time. Not only do you need to be aware of how the workout affects you for the next day or two, but how it might affect your week of training.

You will hear the word split used by runners. This refers to the time it takes to run sections of a race or workout repetition times. Both can yield a lot of information. There are many pacing or split charts available. The times can be used in preparation for and analysis of your performances in both practice sessions and races.

Jim Fischer
Stopwatch
1970s

# Time and Effort

**BRITTANY KELLER**

At the foundation of any solid training is a consistent focus on time and effort. When you see the race champion, a person running so fast while making it appear effortless, or someone you admire for their fitness, it's easy to think they are naturally talented and have something unachievable. I always like to remind the athletes I coach that it's what we don't see that makes them great athletes. What goes unseen is the time and sacrifices they spent training—early morning/lunch hour/late evening runs to reach mileage goals and the planning that goes with it. This is all while juggling their personal lives: school, careers, families, etc.

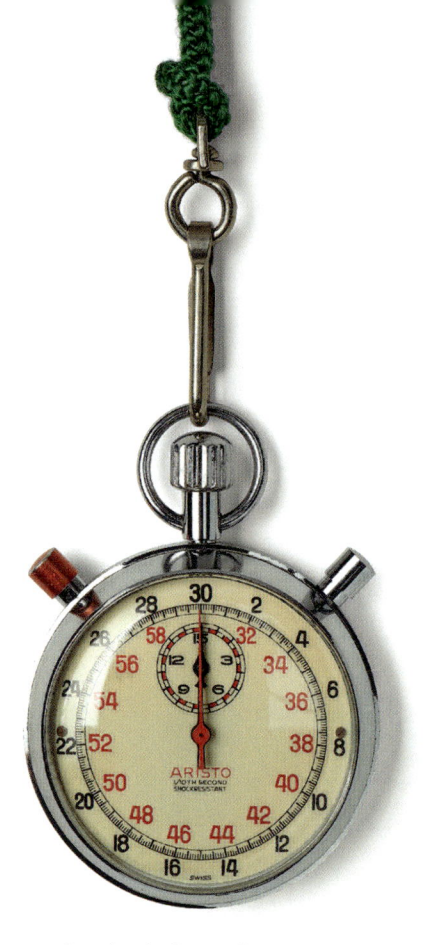

Each individual must figure out how to find the time to make their training possible. While the journey may go unnoticed by others, there's nothing more rewarding than self-reflecting on the hard work, both time and effort, that made your accomplishments possible.

The backstory on the stopwatch pictured: I was given this watch in Spring 2010 during my first year of coaching. I was still in college, preparing to graduate with my undergrad degree. At the time, I had no idea how far me and that watch would go. I thought I would coach for one season. I quickly fell in love

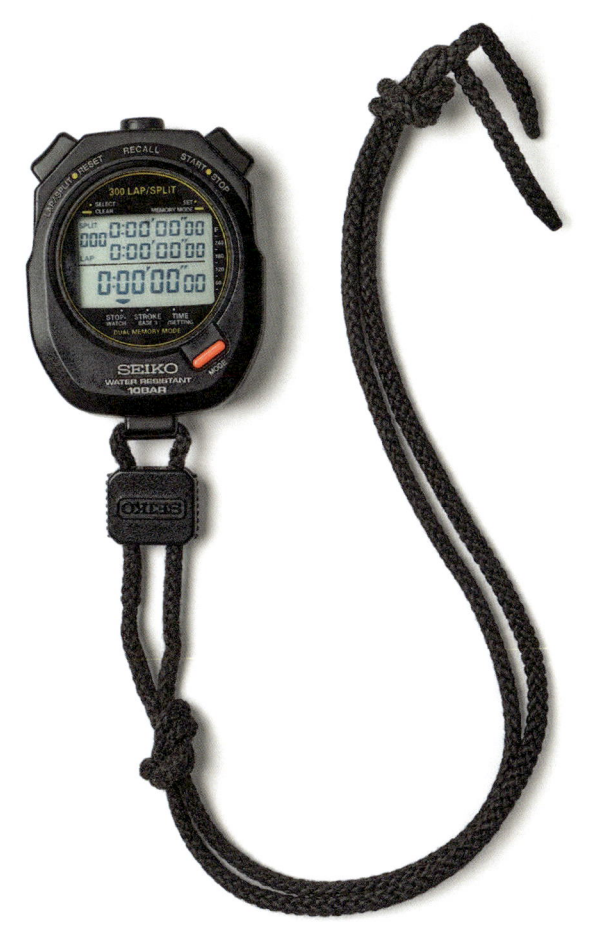

**Brittany Keller**
**Ursuline Academy Coach**
**Stopwatch, 2010-2023**

with coaching and have learned and grown so much over the years, not only from the athletes I've had the pleasure of coaching but also from the coaches I have had the opportunity to coach alongside, especially Jim Fischer and Melanie Aube at Ursuline Academy.

A lot has changed since I was first handed that watch, both in my coaching and personal life. Through it all, one constant has been that watch. Over the years, I've used it to time hundreds of athletes and take thousands of splits. Some were times for beginners in their first race, some were tough losses, some were gritty races, and others were state championship team and individual wins. The emotions include highs, lows, and everything in between. There have been exhilarating and heartbreaking moments, but I wouldn't trade them for anything. All of those memories included me clicking away on that stopwatch. Even though it's getting old and probably should be replaced, I'm hanging on to it as long as I can because it continues to go through my coaching journey with me. After all these years, it's still got a lot left to give, just like me.
Go Raiders, UAXCTF

# Don't write checks your body can't cash.

Coach Art Gulden, Bucknell University

## RECOVERY

Running stresses the body's systems. Time is needed to rebuild all these systems stronger following workouts. There may be times when you decide not to let full recovery happen. Those would be select times and not all the time. You want to teach your body to recover more quickly, but this teaching process takes time. Signs of excess fatigue may include a loss of appetite, weight, energy, enthusiasm, motivation, coordination (which would risk poor body mechanics), power, focus, and concentration.

Additionally, fatigue can cause inefficiency in your running, susceptibility to illness, increased irritability, depression, poor and difficult performances, loss of confidence, elevated heart rate or blood pressure, muscle soreness, and sleeping problems. That's just part of the list. You want to avoid adding dehydration as it hurts the circulation of nutrients, oxygen, blood cells, and fluids for cooling while also slowing the taking of waste products away from cells. One side of the equation is the cooling aspect, perspiration, and evaporation. When body fluids are reduced, there is less fluid for blood, making it thicker and more difficult to pump. The literature suggests that as little as 2% dehydration (2% decline in body weight) can impair performance.

The following diagram illustrates the theoretical ideas of training. It is based on the theoretical model of Nikolai N. Yakovlev developed in the mid-twentieth century. This is simple, yet it conveys the essence of improvement and development. The athlete overloads the system (B to C), and over time, the body must rebuild itself to a higher level, overcompensation (D), to be stronger to withstand more stressful loads in the future.

This is a diagram that can have many outcomes. The horizontal line (A) represents the current fitness level. When a training stimulus (B), a workout, occurs, fatigue sets in (B to C). The workout causes breakdowns in the body, and it needs time to recover (C to D) and build itself stronger than before (A).

## Workout recovery overcompensation model

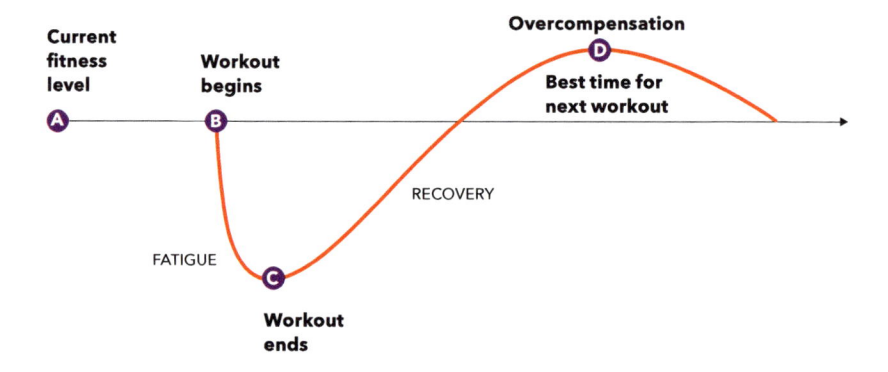

Source: Biochemistry of Sport, N. N. Yakovlev, Leipzig 1967

In the diagram below, if the workout is easier (1), the recovery will be shorter, and the overcompensation peak won't be as high. If the workout is harder (2), the fatigue curve becomes lower, the recovery takes longer, and the overcompensation peak will be higher. The workout (3) may become very tough, going even lower. The recovery may have difficulty returning to the current fitness level, even with a long time to recover. The hope is that the overcompensation peak would be even higher for this hard workout after a very long recovery. Concerns for the runner would be if a strenuous workout would disrupt training, cause excessive fatigue, or bring about an injury or illness.

**Workout intensity model**

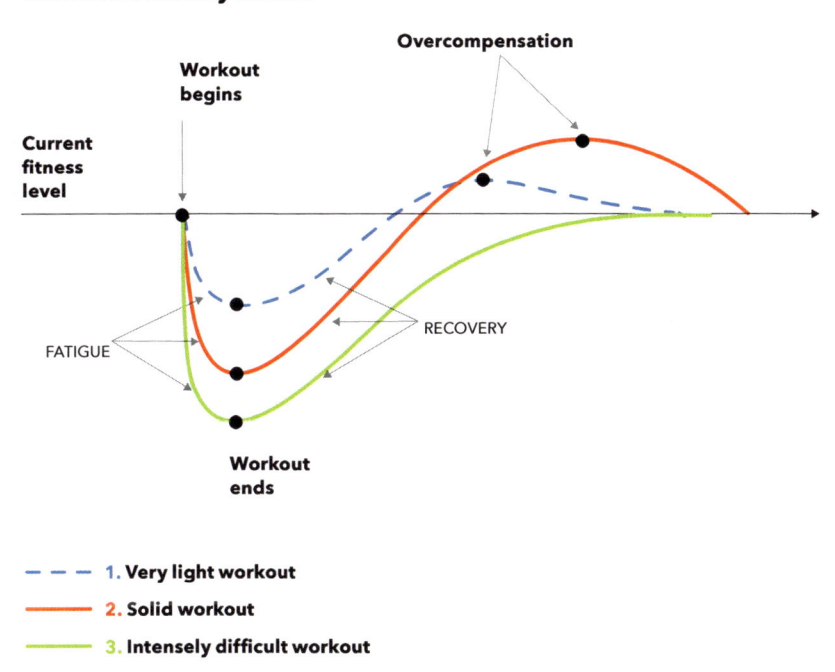

- - - - 1. **Very light workout**
———— 2. **Solid workout**
———— 3. **Intensely difficult workout**

Source: Biochemistry of Sport, N. N. Yakovlev, Leipzig 1967

This goes on as the athlete works to become stronger and stronger. This diagram illustrates the time to introduce the next stimulus, the next hard workout, where the arrow is pointing at the top of the overcompensation peak. A workout causes stress, fatigue, and cell destruction. The body builds itself stronger to withstand the subsequent workout stress better. That means the runner must give the body enough time not only to recover but also to let the body build itself stronger than it was before. If that happens time after time, the athlete will become stronger and stronger, pushing to a higher performance level.

**Ideal workout timing**

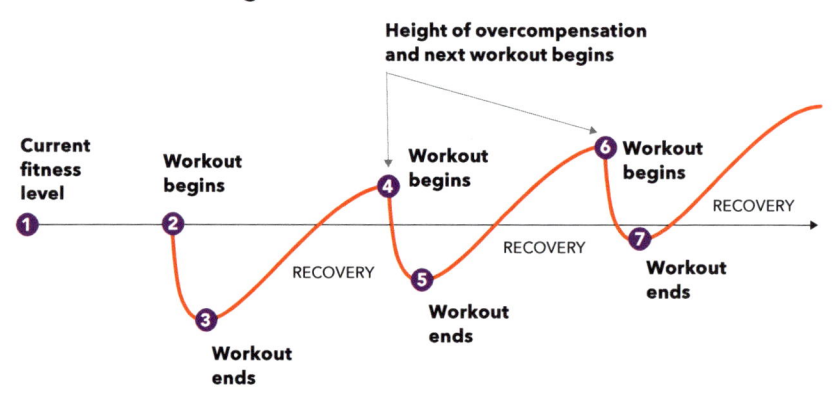

Source: Biochemistry of Sport, N. N. Yakovlev, Leipzig 1967

However, suppose the runner does their next workout too soon before the recovery reaches the original performance level before the body can rebuild itself back to the level it was, let alone get stronger than where it was. In that case, the level of fitness will fail to increase optimally. If this continues to happen often, as the runner doesn't get adequate recovery, the runner will get weaker and weaker, opening the possibility of developing an illness or injury.

If the runner allows a lot of time to go by before doing another workout and waits until the right side of the diagram, where the body is back to the original level of fitness, not only will the person not get stronger, but they'll also lose what they have gained. This is called reversibility; use it, or you lose it. This brings clarity to the training concept.

## Ineffective workout timing

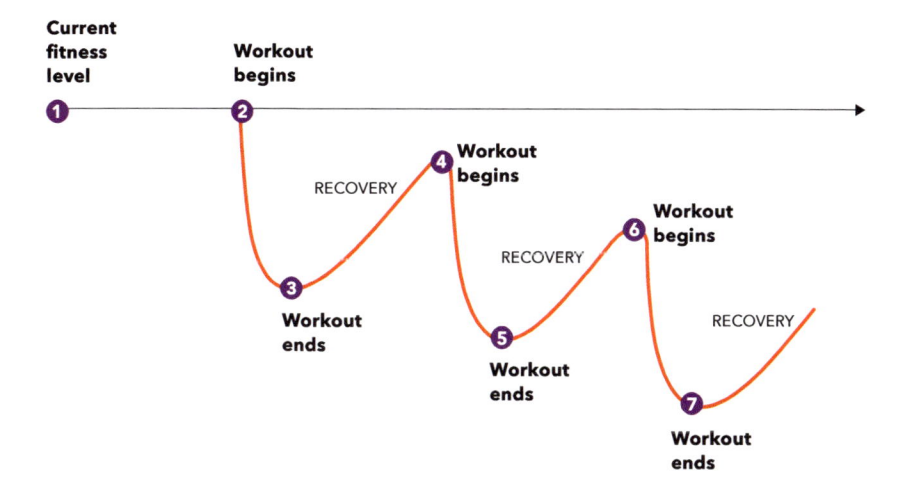

Source: Biochemistry of Sport, N. N. Yakovlev, Leipzig 1967

Recovery from bouts of training is of the utmost importance. Not everyone recovers at the same rate. Years ago, I heard of a world-class athlete with several good training partners, but not at his level. Yet, it took him longer to recover from some of the workouts than it did for his training partners to recover. As strange as that may seem, it emphasizes the point that everyone is different and there is a need to individualize. There may have been things that made the world-class athlete a better racer. Who knows? What is important is that you need to be patient and develop a keen sense of body awareness. You should recover from a workout within the next 24–48 hours. If you are using the hard-easy format, hard one day and easy the next, you should recover from most workouts by the time you are ready for the next hard workout. There are times when you will have to take 72 hours to recover. Early in your training career, you may need to take a day off instead of an easy day. An extra day of recovery may increase the effectiveness of the next training session. Of course, sleep is essential as well. That extra day off may be refreshing, not a day lost in training, but a day gained toward recovery for better training. Overall, manage your fatigue and learn the difference between average daily and chronic fatigue.

There are various strategies to aid in recovery. In addition to good sleep, diet, and hydration, effective methods include stretching, massages, and ice baths. I'll never forget going to an Olympic Trials athlete village and seeing huge ice water baths on the village lawn. Sprinters, middle-distance athletes, distance runners, throwers, jumpers, and vaulters took turns soaking following a workout or competition. This was a part of their recovery and an effort to help prepare them for upcoming competitions.

## MANAGING THE TRAINING CYCLE

When I was a young collegiate coach, we had a team one year that finished second in the conference. They were all underclassmen and returning to run the following year. It was an exciting time. So naturally, the following year, I had the team do the exact same workouts on the very same days. We didn't perform nearly as well as we had the year before. From that, I learned that there is no formula that you can directly apply without considering individual fatigue levels, fitness, progressions in training, and stresses of all kinds— training, academic, family, roommates, social, health, environment, and future life plans. You can't just package things up and automatically assume that there won't be things that will alter plans for attaining goals. Even though I'd always tried to individualize training, it was a lesson that I had to step up my awareness. This leads directly to my caution with generic pre-printed training schedules. These must be viewed as a guide and not as a set of commandments. Everyone in the world doesn't react the same.

Early in your training cycle, the emphasis is on building aerobic endurance while keeping the intensity low. Balance, coordination, speed, strength, and turnover are essential to your training but not the priority now. As the weeks go on and you have developed your endurance fitness to a high level, your training should move toward higher intensity, higher anaerobic fitness, higher quality training, and reaching your goals in races. When the endurance phase feels under control, hills, fartlek, short recovery intervals, tempos, etc., can be introduced.

Balance, coordination, speed, strength, and turnover gain increased importance. In time, the higher intensity phase leads to the main competition part of the training cycle. As the intensity increases, the volume decreases to focus on improving performance. High volume and high intensity are a recipe for fatigue, injury, and illness.

Following the main competition phase, take a few weeks to refresh and rejuvenate before starting your next training cycle. There will be other times when your legs are heavy for a few weeks. No matter what you do, nothing makes them feel better. Back off training for a few weeks and run only when you feel up to it. You will know you are ready to start again when you can't wait to go out for a run.

The level of training you can handle depends upon how old you are, how mature you are physically, mentally, and emotionally, and how long you have been training, in addition to how experienced you are. Someone relatively young in any of these areas should start conservatively with training.

Here, again, is a reminder to keep a log or journal. The journal lets you review your activity for the day and assess what you have done. You will view the day in the context of what you have done in the recent past and allow you to think about what you will do in the short term and long term. You will be able to see what might and might not work for you. You can assess what brings strong results and what might be the root causes of problems.

Let me give an example related to energy, fitness, and health. Let's say that each day, you have a barrel of energy for living, eating, sleeping, studying, working, the environment, relationships, etc. And let's say that you start working hard and do all the activities you need to do in a day. You use up all that day's energy and must begin dipping into the next day's energy supply. As time passes, you take more and more from the next day's supply until that supply is gone, and you must take from two days' supply ahead. This is a recipe for disaster and leads to weakness and increased susceptibility to injury and illness.

## LITTLE THINGS

There was a time in my training when I was trying to run higher mileage than I was accustomed to doing, all the while teaching full-time and coaching. I was squeezing things in. Many days, I was running to and from work. In the morning, I was trying to get as much sleep as possible, run six miles to school, shower, and not be late for class. I always seemed to be cutting it close. I constantly worried about being late and rushed to ensure I would be on time. Trying to run fast to be on time shortly after getting out of bed wasn't working. I was starting to have hamstring issues. Then, I had one of those eureka moments when I figured that if I got up five minutes earlier, I could slow my pace by almost one minute per mile, still be on time, and not have to struggle. It made all the difference in the world. Sometimes, little things count for a lot.

Distance runners who want to improve must be consistent and train even when they don't feel like it. Discipline is an absolutely necessary trait. It separates someone who says they want to get better and someone who really wants to get better. I was at a convenience store near a national cross country championship meet site just after the race was completed. I overheard one of the athletes say that she hadn't had a soda with its empty calories and carbonation all year, and she would finally have one. She had committed that she would do that, among other things, to become the best she could be.

You can view the miles an athlete runs as one of the indicators of their level of fitness. The volume and intensity can be based on the athlete's age, strength, or capacity and their training time. Consider these questions: What must you do to improve your fitness level? Will more mileage make you stronger or injure you? Will higher intensity make you better or produce too much stress?

RUN. TRAIN. RACE.

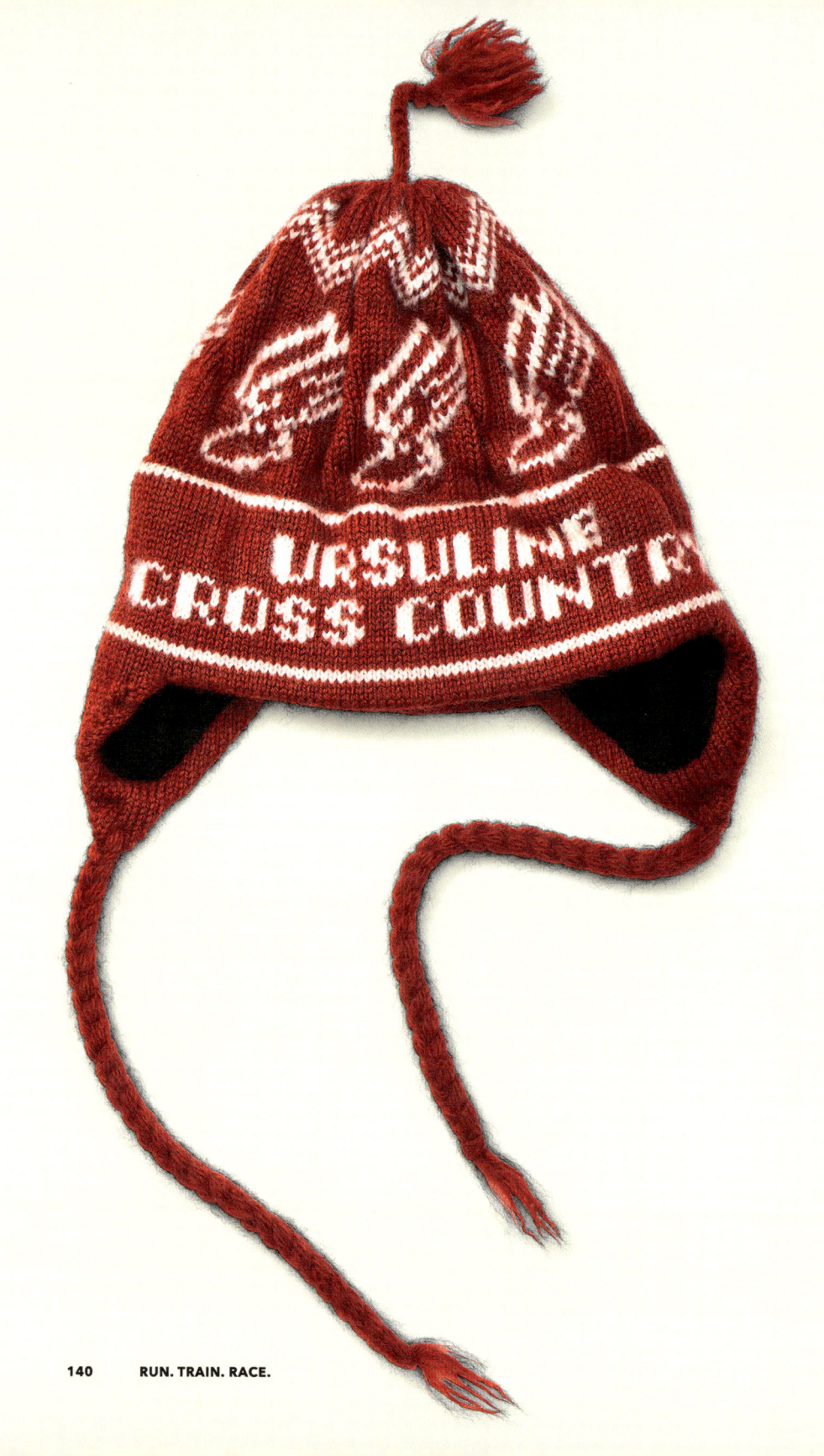

# The Two Things We Can Control

**MELANIE AUBE**

The one thing we always tried to impress upon the girls was the teamwork mentality—always be aware of your teammates' strengths and needs during a race, and know when it's your time to react and step up. Cross Country states at Brandywine Creek in 2018 proved to be a moment when the team truly embraced this principle and found great success. We put two sophomores and five freshmen girls on the line. Each talented in her own right, but also timid and somewhat inexperienced. We knew we could win, but there are always so many variables that unfold during a race. Something magical happened that day. The race didn't unfold as we thought, but the girls reacted and stepped up for one another and unlikely heroes emerged.

They lifted one another and filled gaps to achieve their goal, thus beginning a three year reign as Delaware Girls' Division 2 State Champions! There are two things we can always control when working together as a team—attitude and effort, and on that day, our girls did just that! The chemistry of that team and our coaching staff proved to be very special, and one that was built around the talent, heart and soul of Jim Fischer!

Melanie Aube
Ursuline Academy Coach
UAXC hat, 2012

If you miss a workout, don't try to make it up by doing twice as much the next day. I've also found that many younger athletes need to be "encouraged" to do a full workout, while most collegiate and post-collegiate athletes need control to avoid doing too much. If you considered it an especially important workout, one that would add that little extra to your training or indicate where you are in your training, reschedule it for some time in the future. For the most part, no workout will make all the difference in the world. Therefore, planned, progressive, consistent, and challenging training is critical to your progress. It is the same reason for missing days due to injury or illness. If you are working daily on things that will make you better and have been for a long time, missing days to get healthy will affect you but won't cause you to start all over again. After a few days, you can continue your training to feel better and get your rhythm back. In time you will learn that there are days when you shouldn't run or race and that those days will be positive rather than negative.

There are many ways of doing things that can bring positive results. In daily life, rules of conduct, finance, training, etc., get calm out of commotion and direction out of disarray. Rules provide focus and help guide behavior to meet your goals. I had an athlete who worked extremely hard. We discussed and planned how he could get better and meet his goals. One night, I saw him smoking a cigarette. I was stunned. He worked hard for me in the afternoon and then reversed his gains at night. Do things that help and avoid things that prevent you from achieving your goals.

Acclimatization is essential to perform at a high level regardless of cold, heat, humidity, or altitude. The general rule is that it takes about two weeks to get used to weather factors and a bit longer for altitude, depending on how high. Heat and humidity are the most common factors to deal with. People who don't live in a hot and humid climate have had to make artificial conditions, like wearing extra clothing to prepare themselves for heat and humidity. Living in these conditions usually makes the transition smoother. Dealing with altitude has many challenges, including the early onset of fatigue, altitude sickness, sleep deprivation, dry air, perceived effort changes, and longer recovery. Your maximum speed will also be compromised. The longer you stay at altitude, the more adaptations in your body will make living and training easier. It all takes time.

Don't be afraid to switch directions on a track, especially on an indoor track. If you are always running in the usual direction around a track, counterclockwise, the stresses and torques on the body, especially the legs, will always be the same. Overuse and injury will happen much more frequently. Hopefully, going in the opposite direction around a track sometimes will even out the stresses. If others are simultaneously on the track as you, this may only be possible if you run in one of the outer lanes. Similar problems are associated with running on the same side of the road because of the crown or curvature and with running on a slanted beach. The jarring motions irritate joints, muscles, ligaments, and cartilage and can cause pain and agony.

Many times, it takes work to fit everything into your training schedule. You think you have an enormous amount of time and suddenly realize you don't. Sometimes, it takes minor alterations, such as combining various aspects to cover everything. Determine what things you need to accomplish, how many days each week you will train, how much time you have each day, and set your plan. I prefer to alternate hard and easy running days. Sometimes, I schedule two hard days or two easy days in a row. You may want to work hard two days in a row to force the body to function correctly, even in extreme fatigue. In that case, the first day of training is usually more difficult. You may also want to simulate a track & field meet with trials one day and finals the next to see how you will handle that stress. You should take two or more easy days to ensure you have recovered from a hard workout or race. But generally, the schedule would be a hard day and then an easy day.

With strength work, I alternate work and rest days. You can do your hard strength and running workouts on the same day to make your easy workout days recovery days. But this would make hard days really hard and might compromise the strength work.

At times, I've had my athletes do strength training on their easy running days because we run out of time on the hard training days. Another alternative is to have their strength session in the morning. If you want to, you can do upper body one day and lower body the next or pushing exercises one day and pulling exercises the next. In any case, recovery is essential to make gains!

Do the work in practice that reflects what you want to do in competition. Do some practices at the time of day you will be racing on a surface similar to the competition site in the weather conditions as close as possible to those you will encounter on race day. Simulating everything might be difficult, but get as close as you can. Set up your workouts to practice the demands of the race and strategies you might use or respond to during the competition. The more times you practice these elements, the more comfortable you will feel with them.

As you go through your workouts, week after week, month after month, year after year, your volume and intensity will increase as a natural growth of your training. Sometimes, looking back on the training, you will be surprised by what you could accomplish and what workouts you could do, while when you were doing them, it seemed a natural progression. That's what is supposed to happen!

Get comfortable with being uncomfortable.

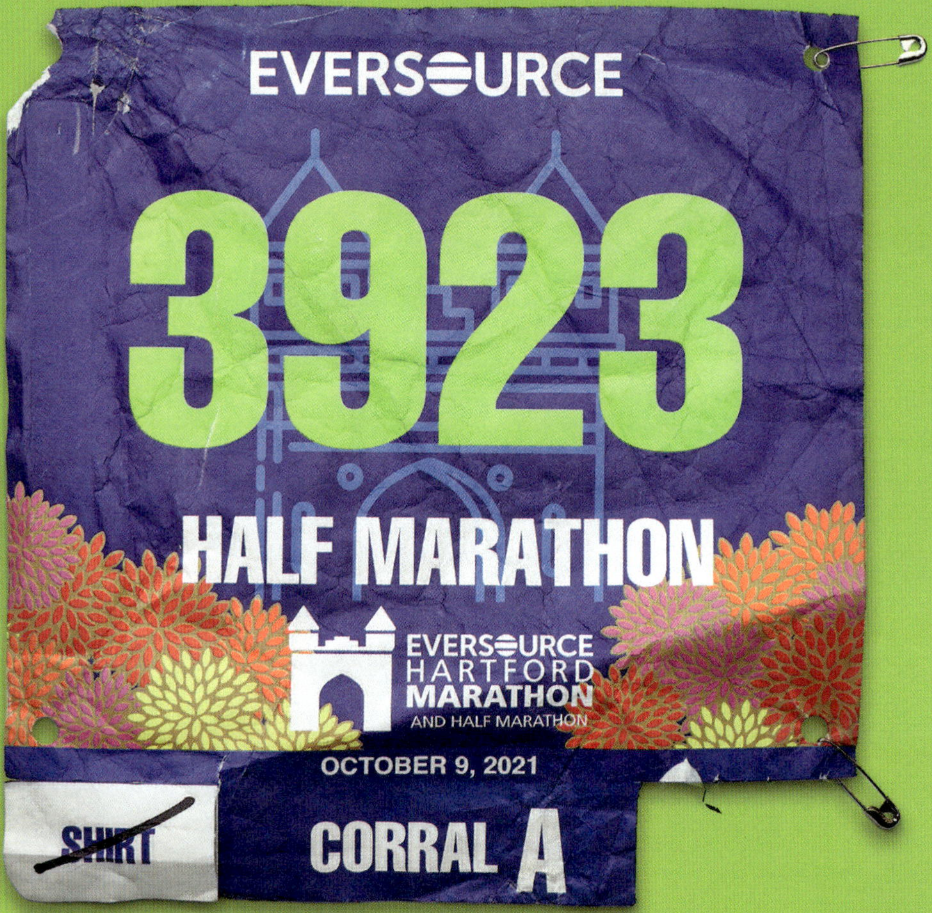
EVERSOURCE
3923
HALF MARATHON
EVERSOURCE
HARTFORD
MARATHON
AND HALF MARATHON
OCTOBER 9, 2021
SHIRT
CORRAL A

# RACE

I wasn't a great runner. But there were people with whom I was competitive in road races. One year, we ran one 15K race with a brutal 800m hill in the middle of the course. In my training for this particular race, I emphasized working on hills, especially the one on the course, so I was comfortable and confident. I had learned a little about visualization techniques, and before the race, I repeated the exercises to train myself to visualize a successful completion of the race. I pushed that hill hard during the race and broke away, and my competitors couldn't catch me. That preparation, plus the visualization of the performance, gave me the feeling that I had been there before.

Laura McMillan
**Race tag**
**Eversource Half Marathon**
Hartford, CT, 2021

## HERE ARE FIVE THINGS THAT WILL HELP YOUR RACING THOUGHT PROCESS

1. Prepare for the specific aspects you need to be successful and get to the race rested and healthy.

2. Personal record times, PRs, are great motivators for racing well! But learn to race to a strategy or against competitors, regardless of the time you get. Sometimes, think about beating people or the course instead of your finishing time. Don't just play defense, responding to what others are doing. Think about going on offense and dictating your strategy.

3. Work on the mental, physical, and emotional aspects that will allow you to respond to your competitors in real-time.

4. You can count many things as "wins" and accomplishments more than just the final results. Think about race strategy successes, positive adjustments made during the race, how a "bad patch" was managed, and the ability to control your rhythm, relaxation, and concentration.

5. Be patient!!!

## THE GOAL

Some people run because they want the activity. Great! Some people run because they like pushing themselves in training and using a race to measure its effectiveness. That's super! Many people want to put themselves into a racing situation because they can test themselves, run with others, or measure themselves against others. I've always said that people from outside the running community have little understanding of the courage it takes to race, and I mean the courage to truly race. I don't say this to demean the other activities, as I've participated in many, and they test me to my fullest. I want everyone to know that runners (racers) deserve equal recognition for their courage.

Racing is about concentration, using different strategies, and dealing with ever-changing circumstances. It takes practice for skills to become instinctive. When one thing doesn't work as planned, you move on to Plan B, Plan C, or Plan D. If you are trying a distance race for the first time or aren't concerned about finishing strong, especially a long-distance race, take walking breaks at regular intervals. Have a plan and stick to it. You want to walk before you are so tired that you are forced to walk. When you have trained and raced for a while and feel ready to be competitive, there are numerous things to consider.

Along with multiple plans for a race, you can have various goals. These goals may concern strategies, feelings, time, place in the field, PRs, records, money, scholarships, qualifying standards, invitations, etc. They could also be performance levels, like your ultimate, secondary, and minimal goals. If it is your first race, the goal is to finish feeling good.

Most everyone needs to learn how to race. It isn't a natural thing for most people. It takes a while to get used to the feeling of a race effort. That's why you need to practice racing. A race can be a "quiz" leading to a significant "test" later. Learn to control the pace at the start of the race, even if you are going hard from the starting gun. Don't let emotions carry you away. The goal is to learn to anticipate the strategic moves of others and set up your moves, whether you are responding to others, which is a defensive strategy, or creating and controlling your offensive tactics. With experience, you will instinctively learn to anticipate and identify things happening during a race, which will help you to become more successful.

Racing is part of the training process. Not every race is the most important race of the month, the season, or the year. There are goal races that you work toward, but races can be used as workouts, different race strategies, race day preparations, simulations for longer races, working with and helping others, and so on. Races early in the season are developmental, preparing you for the goal race(s). Use them to support your training and fitness. In those races, practice a fast race start, a slow race start, an even pace race, etc. You can pace another slower runner and help them with their race effort. You can run to support a charity or for social reasons. You can learn to schedule your pre-race meals, hydration, registration, bathroom visits, and warmup. You can learn to control your emotions and keep yourself relaxed. You want to have all of this figured out by the time you get to your big race so you aren't guessing. Nevertheless, you should prepare for every race and be ready when the gun goes off.

Some people love to race. They love the challenge and the opportunity to learn where they are in their training and to be able to show others the product of their work. For some, head-to-head competition is more important than time or records. Others love to train and work on their fitness but get incredibly nervous about racing. Nervousness can stem from the athlete's concern that they may not meet their expectations. They may be concerned about the pain involved in completing the race. The expectations of others may bother some runners. For some, the only reason they run is to be social. For those apprehensive about racing, I suggest that they change things up to keep it fresh. Try doing a destination race, tying it to going somewhere fun. Or do just the opposite. Set certain local races as annual events where you know people and have time to see them afterward. It might be an opportunity to have family and friends watch you compete. Or you can tie yourself to run with someone slower than you to take the pressure off. You could also try setting an easy goal to gain some confidence.

How many races should you run? The answer to this question varies widely. Some people will race in only a few select races. They focus on training and direct their energy on those limited efforts. The danger here is that running at race level differs from training level, and it can become challenging to maintain interest and focus. They may need more practice with race tactics, strategy, situational recognition, and the toughness required to become proficient. Other people run in many races. They enjoy the frequent challenges and the social aspects. Problems with overuse injuries, energy depletion, staleness and "dead" legs, limited training outside of races, and lack of focus on one main event may prevent them from reaching their true potential. If you want to race well, you need to practice a variety of racing situations, whether in practice or actual races, so that you can learn to race instinctively. It's great to experience as many situations as possible to learn how to respond. However, it is important not to race so much that it limits your ability to focus on the big race or the amount of training required to be successful.

## PACING, PACING, PACING

Most people learn their pace using a stopwatch and consulting a pace chart when needed. That's fine. A stopwatch has its place. Work toward learning to feel your pace without using a watch. Let's say you are running a 5K and get to the one-mile mark too fast or too slow. At the one-mile mark, it's probably already too late for you to meet your goal time because if you were too fast, the end could be ugly, and if you were too slow, you might have already lost a lot of time.

There are good reasons to start fast. You want to push your limits, you want to run with the leaders as long as you can, you want to place in the race or your age group, or you want to run a fast time. These are all excellent reasons. If you are too fast, it may be a struggle to finish. You burn carbohydrates and build lactic acid faster than you can eliminate it. Somewhere near the end of the second mile of a 5K, the burning and pain will take command of your body, and the rest of the way won't be fun. Remember that going out hard in a long-distance road race differs from going out hard for a mile on the track. If it is a longer race, the "won't be fun" part will last a long time.

People need to realize that running too slow, while usually not as painful, will also get in the way of your goal. Let me give an example. Let's say you go to a racetrack that is two miles long, and you will drive your car at 60 miles per hour around the track in the first trial. How long does it take you? Two minutes, right? Next, you will drive your car around the track again, driving the first mile at 30 miles per hour. How fast do you drive your car the second mile to finish in two minutes, the same as you finished the first trial? Do you have the answer? The 30 miles per hour you drove for the first mile already used up the two minutes. No matter how fast you went the second mile, you still wouldn't finish in two minutes. Time spent is time you can't get back.

I'm often reminded of pacing when I watch a two-mile or 5K distance race for youth or high school athletes. Invariably, a few runners will start extremely fast for the first 400m, jog most of the race, then 200m from the finish run a strong sprint through the finish line to the crowd's amazement. I like to tell runners that they probably saved five seconds over the last 200m, whereas if they had distributed that energy during the rest of the race, they might have saved 30 seconds or more.

This involves your energy and comfort level. There is a level of discomfort or pain that you must endure, and if you are going to run at a faster pace, that level will be higher. The higher your pain tolerance, to an extent, the faster you can run throughout the race. You may not have a blazing finish, but you might be competing against a different level of runners. Fast racers aren't always the people who are the most talented. They might be the people who can and will tolerate the most pain.

There are many occasions when you should use an even-paced strategy or run a negative split, a race in which you run faster during the second half. Some examples of when you might do this are early in the racing season when you are low in confidence because you are unsure if you are ready to race, you are nervous, you are exhausted, you currently have a slight injury or illness, you have had an injury or illness and want to get back into a race, your fitness level is low, you feel weak, you want a solid effort in preparation for future training and racing, or the weather conditions aren't optimal such as running in hot and humid weather. Early in the racing season, give yourself a break by running a controlled effort as a preliminary to building into your more critical races.

Many race strategies, from simple to very complex, can be used for races of all distances. Some may be more appropriate for some distances, but a case can be made for using almost anything in any race. Almost everyone develops their favorite race strategy and uses it most of the time. Limiting yourself to the same strategy all the time may keep you from developing some aspects of your fitness and racing ability. Someone else employing a completely different strategy you have never used could be unsettling and hurt your performance.

## RACING AS A PART OF THE TRAINING CYCLE

Racing times take a while to catch up to workout performances and projections, which can be challenging to comprehend. Sometimes, the lag time can be six months to a year. The reasons can be physiological, psychological, or a lack of confidence. Be patient, not only with race times but also with workouts. If you are doing the work and doing it correctly, good things will happen.

Travis Adams
UD athlete 1990-1995
Adidas 'Tech Star LD'
racing spikes, 1994

# Race Day Jitters

**TRAVIS ADAMS**

Packing a bag—singlet and shorts, spikes and wrenches, tape, sweats. Hat and gloves? Or extra T-shirts? Prepare for all weather! Finding a home base, get set up in the stands, double check everything. Are we on time, or running behind? Warming up, easy at first then harder. Review the race plan—what are the goals, who am I running with, and against?

Focus inward. Last minutes—uniform on, yellow spikes tied tight and double-knotted, strides to work out the last jitters.

And then after so few minutes, it's over. Hours and weeks and months of preparation for such short bursts of absurd effort! During the races I remember bits of the race strategy,

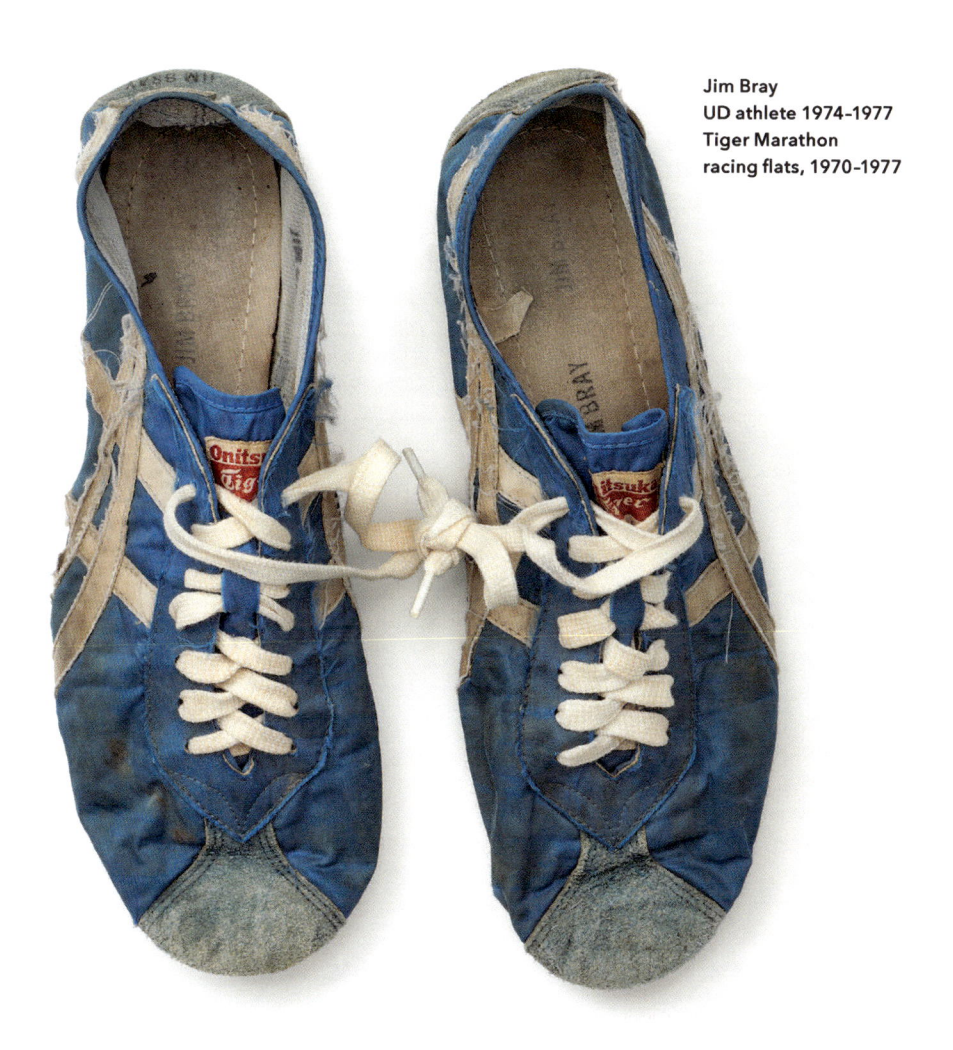

Jim Bray
UD athlete 1974–1977
Tiger Marathon
racing flats, 1970–1977

the splits, the jostling or the efforts to stay in contact or break away. In the best races, the focus lasts from the starter's gun to the finish.

Looking back over decades, these spikes remind me of those efforts mostly in the context of the numbers associated with the races. 15:00 (and a 1–2 finish!) on a banked oval.

14:31.03 (last place after a lap, but a 31-second closing 200m) at a truly historic meet. 30:19.77 (so close to a school record but never approached again). And oddly, only the place and not the time of the only conference race I ever won. I was lucky to compete in all of them.

RUN. TRAIN. **RACE.** 155

Peaking, being at your absolute best on your goal race day, is about preparation. Tapering your training as you approach a goal race lets the body build itself back up after much hard work. Cut back on your total mileage during the taper or the recovery period leading to your goal race. The better-conditioned you are, the longer you can maintain peak performance. As I stated earlier, the last major workout should be about eight to ten days before the most important race. Maintain hard work, but reduce the volume overall. Do fast-paced but shorter workouts to stay in touch with your turnover and speed but controlled at a decreased total volume. You can't do much to help yourself in those last few days, but you can do things that can hurt. Prepare to feel good and run well.

Signs that you are ready for your big race: quick recovery rate, motivated and alert, energetic, confident, and excited. Signs that things aren't going well: sick, sore, stiff, tired, irritable, fatigued, depressed, tense, and poor sleeping patterns. Also, remember that when your activity level drops, be aware of the volume of food being consumed. Loading for a long-distance race is one thing. You can accomplish this by eating healthy meals without gorging yourself. Eating the same amount with less total running may make you feel heavy. Hydrate and eat a racing diet for three days before the race. It isn't necessary to load up on carbohydrates more than usual for races under 40 minutes in length. Loading for a mile race will make you feel heavy. For every gram of carbohydrate you eat, three to four grams of water are connected to it. That's a lot of weight. It is a great thing for long races. For short races, not so much!

Practicing pacing and strategy will help you identify your strengths and weaknesses. Knowing who you are running against and their strengths and weaknesses will help. Sometimes, you need luck, but putting yourself in a good position will help. Try to take as many of the variables out of the process. Use race modeling to simulate a race in practice. Do some workouts to simulate the stresses you encounter during the race. That doesn't mean you should run the race in these workouts, even though time trials can be a part of your training. Break down the components into controllable parts to learn what you will face. This is done to give you confidence that you have already faced these situations in practice and understand what to do. One thing to consider when running or watching the end of a race is whether the person getting passed at the end had a bad "kick" or ran at a higher level during the whole race, enduring more pain for an extended period, cutting many seconds off their time, and finishing with all the energy they had left.

## BEFORE THE RACE

I was always nervous before races. I often thought I would fail and have the worst race of my life, no matter how much preparation I'd done. If I lowered my expectations, I would take some pressure off my performance. I hated days when the weather was perfect because I had no excuses. As time went on with my running and coaching, I worked hard with my athletes and myself to think about changing nervousness (negative) to excitement (positive). I wanted everyone to talk themselves into a great performance rather than out of one. I tried to have everyone eliminate "negative speak" and think confidently about the upcoming competition, whether competing against their own goals or racing others.

When I was coaching at Ursuline Academy with Melanie Aube and Brittany Keller, we wanted our athletes to build self-confidence. We had a very young team who were talented and hard-working. But we had to get used to the idea that we were good enough to beat people. We stressed the importance of believing in the process, that the training prepared us for the race, and that running with a team mentality resulted in better outcomes. We were building a winning culture. We came up with the acronym GUTI, which meant Get Used To It. To athlete Laini McGonigle, this meant getting used to grinding out tough

# The Impact of a Great Coach

**PATRICK CASTAGNO**

I have had the great fortune to be involved in the sports of cross country and track & field for over 50 years. I began as a 2nd grader running the 50-yard dash at Baynard Stadium only minutes after eating a hotdog and ended my time on the track as a collegiate miler at the University of Delaware's Track & Field program—with many miles between the two. For the last 23 years, I have taken seriously the responsibility I have been given as a high school cross country and track coach.

Like many, this sport has defined the direction of my life. My eventual life passions began as interesting possibilities suggested by the leaders of my life: famous people, parents, teachers, and coaches. I quickly learned that we are all products of our environment as impressionable youth and that the presence of great leadership in your life can influence you to reach your God-given potential through caring and constant guidance into the process of dreaming big. I hit the jackpot with those who created these strong and supportive environments for me. My coaches and teachers were incredible examples of effective leadership. My high school coach, Father Joseph Beattie, led by inspired actions that got us to believe that all things were possible. My college coach, Jim Fischer, led by example in everything he did. He demonstrated, every day, a thoughtful and respectful interaction with every athlete. He taught us how to think and how to relax when stressed on the starting line. He created an environment where everyone felt welcome and at home on his teams and reminded us to enjoy the journey along the way. Coach's athletes admired and respected him and wanted to impress him. I'm one of so many Jim Fischer athletes who entered the teaching and coaching profession because of the incredible experience and strong influence he had on us as a leader. He changed the direction of our lives.

The power of being a leader is more about empowering others to believe in themselves to take ownership of their own destiny. All great teams or organizations in history have always had strong leadership. As much as we realize great leadership wins team championships, it is also known that poor leadership can ruin a team, business, and even a school.

A leader is someone who has the influence to change the trajectory of a group through their guidance, persuasiveness, and ability to see the future. Being able to see the future is not some psychic power but more about knowing what the next best move to make for the group long before it needs to be made.

Patrick Castagno
Tatnall School Coach
UD athlete 1983–1988
University of Delaware
Track & Field T-shirt
1983

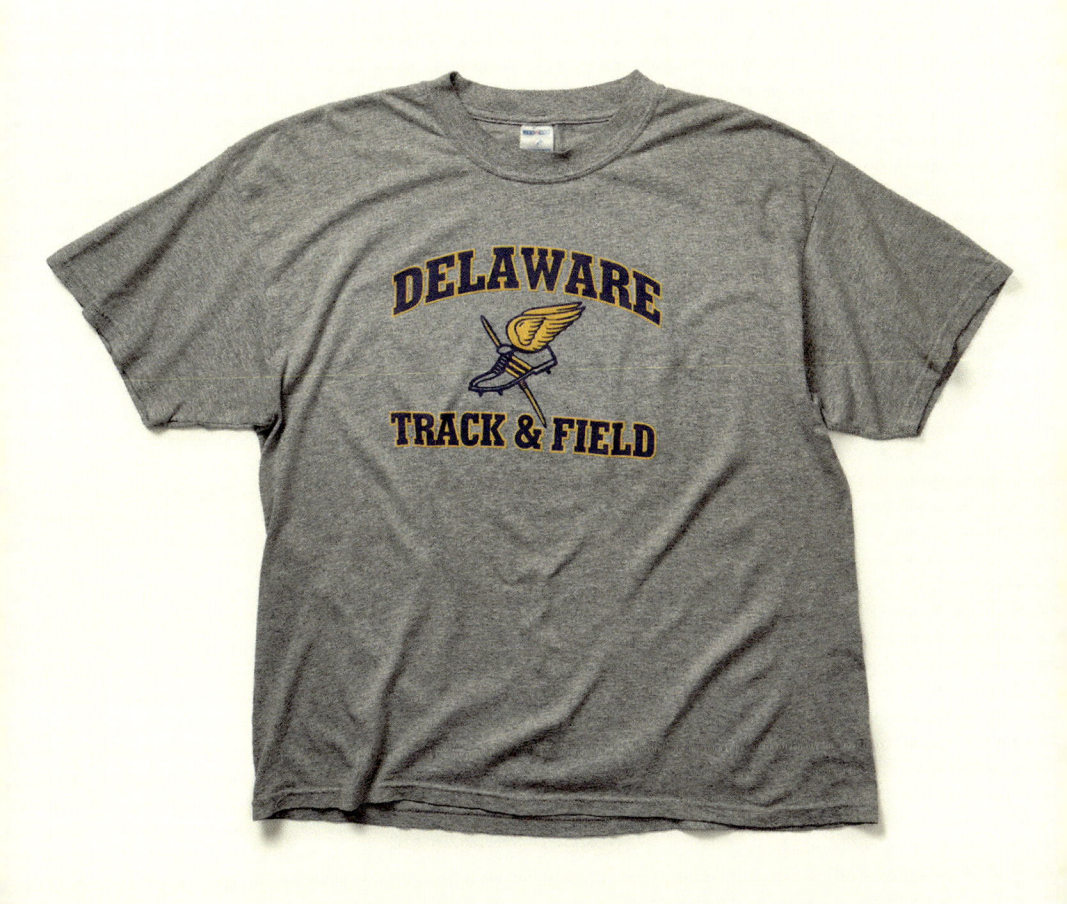

I have been so fortunate, even lucky, to have been around so many great leaders growing up. The result of my experiences under great leadership left me wondering how I could do for others what my coaches did for me and what a fulfilling life that would be.

RUN. TRAIN. **RACE.**

runs and workouts on hot summer days leading up to the cross country season. Get used to being uncomfortable and pushing past that feeling to reach that next level. Get used to working as a team during a race. Get used to leading a race, and most importantly, get used to winning and having confidence. GUTI was also our shorthand for reminding each other that becoming state champions was attainable and what we expected of each other, which became critical in the dark and lonely moments of a tough race. She took this with her as her running career continued in college, battling injuries and fully embracing the grind of working herself back into shape. More importantly, these lessons helped her in other parts of her life, tapping into the mental and physical toughness instilled in her as a runner when she needed to push past her comfort zone and reach that next level.

If you like to have music for your pre-race preparation, find music that suits you. It might be your favorite feel-good tunes. You could also find music that helps control your mood. You might be wired, nervous, or unable to concentrate and need calming and soothing music. Or you could be low-key and calm and need to get fired up with some head-banging music. This is another thing that can be tried in practices or developmental races to find out what is the best for you.

There is no substitute for intense physical and strategic situational preparation. That should help build confidence. Mental, emotional, and psychological preparation are needed as well. Many articles, books, and lectures have addressed visualization—having the athlete see themselves complete successful trials and performances repeatedly in their mind, talking themselves into attaining the desired outcome. It is a mental rehearsal of success for success. This positive approach should be practiced lying down in a relaxed atmosphere with eyes closed and relaxed breathing where it is quiet, dark, and comfortable with no distractions. Visualization, the mindful seeing of one's successful performances, can be practiced daily for a few minutes or many. Vicki Huber-Rudawsky, a two-time Olympian, said she had sessions over an hour reinforcing those positive mental outcomes. This supplements all

It's easy to
find people who
want to win.
It's hard to find
people who
don't want to lose!

the hard work. Visualization enhances it by playing a positive video loop in the head of the athlete, successfully promoting confidence. The goal is for the mind to see success over and over again. The race has already been run. Now, the athlete just has to get to the starting line for the body to complete what has already been seen.

The warmup for a race is essential. I can't tell you the number of people who told me it took them a mile to get warmed up in a race. That may be okay if it is a half-marathon or marathon and you only want to finish or if you are running for fitness or social reasons. If it is a 5K, you are already finished with one-third of your race before you are ready to go. The amount of conditioning you do weekly plays into this. If you want to do well, think of the warmup differently. You must be in good enough shape so that a two-, three-, or even four-mile warmup would enhance your race, not destroy it. There are times when many have told me that they finally got into a good rhythm seven miles into their long run. That should start to tell them something. If you want to race a 5K well and need to keep your warmup short, you will compromise your performance until you get stronger.

## START

At the starting line, especially in a closely bunched track race, tenths of seconds may mean the difference between getting out quickly and running free and clear or having many people ahead with you, just trying to stay upright. Get into your starting position, one foot in front of the other, balanced, with your opposite arm forward. Step quickly and firmly with your back leg when the gun goes off. If you take a short step with your front foot first, you gain little distance, and it will waste valuable time for your positioning.

To start a race, especially a long one, ensure you stay true to your plan. Have practiced starts enough so you know what to expect. Don't let your emotions cause you to run faster than planned. Don't panic. All those people sprinting past you at the start are either people who will come back to you later or can maintain that pace, and you may have trouble beating them anyway. They generally don't give out medals at the halfway point in the race. Focus on you and your plan! Run tall and relaxed with a good rhythm, especially as the race goes on when you start to fatigue.

## IN THE RACE

When you are in a race, here is a checklist: relaxation, pace, race position and strategy, form, rhythm, and easy, even breathing. You especially need to think about these things when you are tired. Keep your head level and your eyes up unless footing is a problem. Don't look back. Instead, focus on catching the person ahead of you. That doesn't mean you can't look back to be aware of who is behind you. However, some constantly look back, interrupting their focus on what is ahead. Assume that someone is behind you and will attempt to pass you at the end of the race. Go hard through the finish. Some other things you can think about to mix things up a little are taking risks to test fitness, thinking of strategy to block you from thinking of the pain, learning what to do from different positions in the pack, working toward the next runner, looking at the runner's shoulders and not their feet, running over the top of hills, surging and learning when to and when not to use it, paying attention to other runners' breathing, and relaxing and getting into a natural rhythm to fight off a "bad patch" mid-race. This list isn't all-inclusive.

In elite-level racing, with everyone at approximately the same ability and fitness, losing concentration for even 100m may be problematic. It could be enough for the runner to lose contact with the athletes they had been running with. They may lose their ability to get back with the group before the end of the race. Also, for anyone, loss of concentration in the middle of the race, usually just after the halfway mark, can derail even the best of efforts. Keep your rhythm and stay engaged in the task at hand. This is the same for all of us. It requires training to learn how to relax and stay focused on what you are doing. Practice this during your workouts.

Strategy, figuring out how fast you can run, and determining who you should be running with are aspects of racing that must be practiced. An evenly paced plan is the most efficient way to race but may never lead you to explore your potential. Try going out fast a few times. It's a great way to test your limits when you are ready for it. Can you physically and psychologically break from the field? How fast can you go, and how long can you hold it? Will your energy run out before the race does? Do you trust your conditioning? Can you run strongly enough to carry it on to the finish? Can you go a little farther each race at this faster pace? Can you "settle in" to a pace after a while so that you can respond when you are challenged again, especially near the end of the race?

Or should you go out slowly? The danger with this strategy is that people may get away from you, and you might not see them again until the post-race refreshments. If you start too slowly, will you be able to get back to the athletes you know you can be competitive with? Will your ability to pass runners later in the race get you close enough to be competitive? Will you dig yourself such a big hole that you won't be able to climb out of it before the finish? Will you get discouraged or get "stuck" in the slower pace and stay slow, unable to work your way back? There are many more questions.

My first "go-to" standard for race strategy is one that I borrowed. It isn't the only strategy I've used, but the basic one I almost always start with. I attended a panel where the term "critical zone" was discussed. This is like football, which uses the term "red zone" to highlight the part of the field where success is critical. The ability of a football team to determine a way to be successful when it is near the goal line defines the team's character. In distance running, the first two-thirds to three-fourths of the race is about getting a good tactical position, staying relaxed and controlled, and using as little energy as possible.

You don't have to run slowly. If you can stay relaxed while letting others do the pace work and break the wind, that will set you up for a strong finish. It is hard, but be patient.

This doesn't mean you can't lead or help dictate the race's strategy. It means that if you use a lot of energy getting to the two-thirds to three-fourths mark of the race, you probably won't have the energy to respond to someone else's surge to the finish. Make sure to maintain your concentration between the halfway point and the start of the critical zone, a troublesome time in a race for many runners as their pace tends to lag. I like to define the critical zone as the last third of the race to be more intentional for this challenging period just after halfway. Commit most of your energy and focus to the critical zone. It is more fun to pass people at the end of a race rather than being passed. It gives such a mental lift. Be confident, in control, and ready to move. Practice "owning" the end of the race. So again, start the race, establish your position, maintain a good pace and rhythm, use as little energy as possible, and go hard the last third of the race.

This strategy is directly applicable to many situations. It is particularly valuable in longer races. If you go out too hard in a marathon, or even a 5K or 10K, you are going to use carbohydrates as the primary fuel, your core temperature will increase, you will lose water and salts more rapidly, and the acid build-up in the muscles will affect your performance. It is like a race between the inside of your body and the outside race that you are trying to finish with a strong performance. Will your carbohydrates run out? Will your core temperature go too high, inhibiting your performance? Will you have enough water to cool and efficiently fuel your body with enough electrolytes to function correctly? Will the acid buildup limit your muscle function? Which side will win that race?

When learning to run in a tight group, practice running in all positions. Try running in front, in back, on the sides, and in the middle. Find a comfort level in all places. You may have a favorite strategy or way to

Vicki Huber-Rudawsky
Eight-time NCCA champion
and two-time Olympian
US Olympic team jacket
Atlanta, GA, 1996

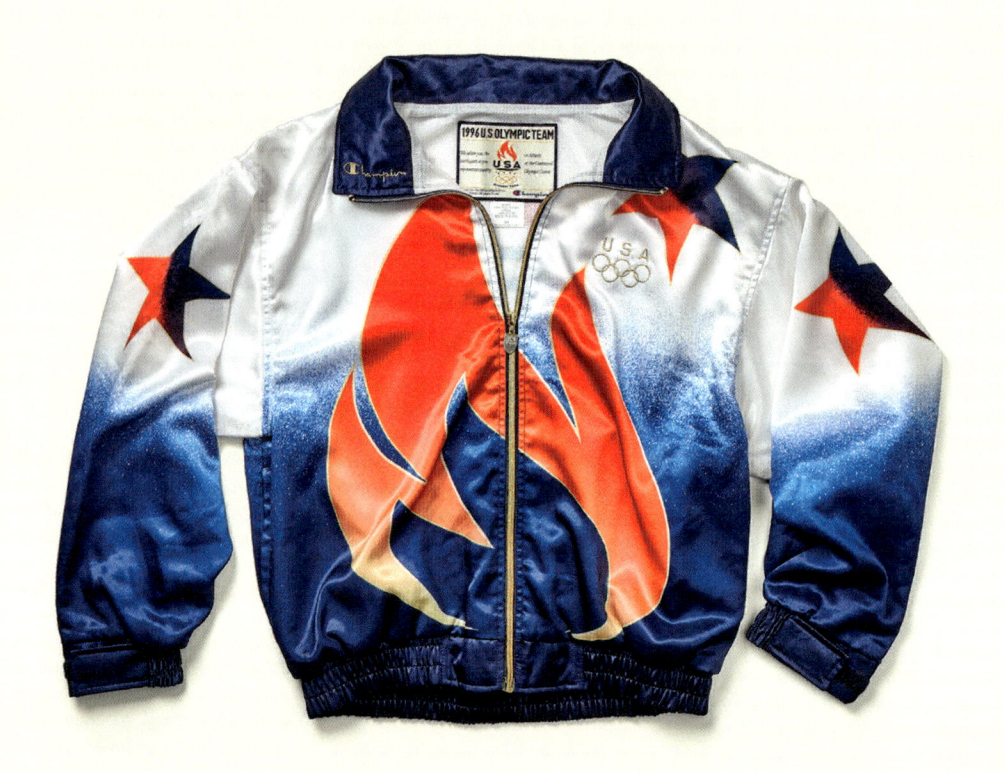

# One Random Meeting

**VICKI HUBER-RUDAWSKY**

After dropping out of the 5000m with less than two laps to go, and in perfect position to make the final, I was devastated. And embarrassed. Although I knew deep inside that for whatever reason, it was the right thing to do, it was still confusing and I didn't know how to respond to people.

I was in the position to come back and run the 1500m, since I had met the qualifying times for both, and there were a few days between the races to recuperate. I had called and cried to my friend Kris out in Oregon, and she just told me to do what had worked for me in every situation—pray. I also had a sore left foot, so a day or two after the disaster in the 5000m, I went for a run on the roads of Dunwoody, GA to test my foot and to think—I was not staying where most of the athletes were because my daughter and parents were with me, so I figured I wouldn't see anybody I didn't want to see on the short run.

As I ran, I soon saw a figure running towards me in the distance. I remember thinking, "Oh crap. I didn't want to see anybody. I hope they don't recognize me." As the figure approached, I realized the runner was Coach Fischer. I am sure we were both surprised and amazed to see each other on the random streets of Dunwoody! We stopped for a few minutes to chat, and what I remember most is that Coach didn't ask me what happened, or why I dropped out. All he said was, "How are you?"

That random meeting, I now know, was meant to be. I turned around to run back to the house knowing that I was going to run the 1500m, if not for any other reason than to prove to myself that I was not a quitter or a loser. I was the last person to make it out of each of the two qualifying heats, and ultimately finished third in the finals to make the Olympic Team.

As anyone who knows Coach knows, his kind and gentle person was just what I needed that day. There was no judgment, no criticism, but also no pity. He was the push to remember who I was.

race, but you also may be thrust into any of these situations, and you must be able to relax and be confident. Some runners are very comfortable leading a group. They want control and are willing to spend their physical and psychological energy to lead and break the wind for the rest to have control. Others stay in the back, just being towed along for the ride. Using the group as shelter from the wind is a great reason to stay behind others. In a pack where things are a little crowded, refrain from darting back and forth to find free space, essentially unnecessarily doing an interval workout and using a lot of energy. Be patient and see if things open up so you can move to free yourself from a boxed-in position. You can gradually move your positioning so that the people around you have to make decisions about their position, which may help things open up. If the race is short, you may force the decision more aggressively.

Most people find it best to run next to someone, just off their shoulder and slightly behind. While running directly behind a runner, there are the potential problems of bumping legs, getting spiked, or stepping on a heel. Watching the movement of their legs gave me the illusion that they were running away from me and certainly running faster than me. By running next to and slightly behind, I could use their shoulder as a frame of reference, which most people didn't move very much. It meant that I could keep my head up. This was especially helpful if I was starting to struggle. It was a little chance to relax and refocus.

Be strong and be aware of what is happening around you. Watch others and listen to their breathing. Determine who is struggling and who isn't. Pay attention. A problem can arise if you aren't alert when runners in the front positions accelerate and make a break from the rest of the group. This is especially a problem if you are in the middle, have nowhere to go, and can't make a move to go with the front runners. Pay attention! If the runners are all of equal ability, five meters may be enough of a lead that you won't catch them before the end of the race. The middle of the pack can also be treacherous, with arms and legs going in every direction. Tangled legs aren't fun. It is a good place if everyone is calm. If people are jumpy, darting in and out, or unsteady with their pacing, it can make the middle a scary place. Staying on the outside shoulder slightly behind the leader gives you the advantage of being able to move when you want. You might catch some wind but can put yourself in a strong position.

Learn to stay in contact with a group or another runner. Don't even give them a meter of space. If you can't be that close physically, keep mental contact to somehow tie you to them. They are the connection between you and the other athletes in the race. They help you focus on working your way back up to them to be competitive with everyone else. The focus should be on bridging the gap and returning to direct contact. Some people prefer to run a race with no one around them. That isn't what most people want. Most want to run with another individual or a group. In cases where you find yourself in no man's land with no one around you, work your way to the next group, latch onto them, and then take a little breather from the work you just did. If there is no group close to you, relax and concentrate on keeping your rhythm.

If you have been gapped and have a distance to make up to catch the next person, focus with your eyes up and on them. Try not to let that gap open in the first place. But if it does, change your rhythm to get back up to them. "Throw them a rope" and gradually work your way back to the group. Look at them. Stay in mental contact. Constantly work toward getting up to the next person and the next. Concentrate on their singlet and will yourself back to them. When you get back up to them, settle in for a few seconds to catch your breath, relax, and recover. It is frustrating if they decide to speed up at the same time as you do or increase their pace just when you have gotten back in contact. That's a risk you will have to take.

When mirroring someone's rhythm, pay attention that they don't slow without you noticing. Don't get lulled to sleep thinking you are maintaining a good pace. That can negate the good work that you have done. Pass another runner quickly to open distance and break their will. When being passed, change your rhythm to go with them. Pay attention to other runners. Is their breathing strained? Are they struggling? How are their form and foot strike? Are they relaxed? If they are having trouble, can you take advantage? Anticipate an upcoming hill, a turn, bad footing, a group up ahead, or someone trying to pass you that might cause you to be boxed in. Surging may allow you to break from a group, give a clear view of the course or track, or charge up a hill, but there are costs. Practicing will help you understand the costs and the competitive risks involved.

A strong, steady rhythm is great. There are times when you want to get "stuck" in that rhythm, and there are times when you don't—when getting "stuck" means you will fall farther and farther behind. When you get tired, try to maintain your rhythm unless your pace is rapidly decreasing. Getting into a solid rhythm can be a very efficient way to cover a lot of ground. But if your stride length, stride frequency, or both deteriorate when you get tired, it can cause you to slow dramatically. When this happens, shorten your stride instead of trying to lengthen it. You can also try to quicken your rhythm to catch someone or ward off a challenge. Sometimes, you might lose your concentration. Changing rhythm can help you regain focus and revitalize your race effort. Do anything to stay focused and engaged. Road and cross country races can do this automatically for you with hills, turns, predetermined strategy, surges, and competitor or personal challenges. In fact, on some courses, constantly changing rhythms is the norm. All this needs to be practiced.

Surging, pushing the pace for short sections during a race, is a great tactic, especially if you are equal to or better than the competition. However, it can be used to your advantage even if you aren't. It must be practiced, or it could lead to your disaster. Going hard from the beginning can take people by surprise. You can use it to "soften" your competitors. If you want to pass someone, if the pace is controlled, make the pass quickly and carry it on to open a gap. Be careful. It may doom you later if you make an extremely hard surge or pass.

When you know other runners are always extremely fast at the finish, you might start the race harder than usual, attack a hill or another part of the course, or drive to the finish line from farther away to neutralize your opponents' late speed. A surge as you approach the finish area can help you make it difficult for someone to catch you. If you have practiced and are ready, this could come from a long way out. Surges can be planned or a reaction to something that has happened. Be aware that you might have one or two opportunities to have the energy to make a major move, so you want to use them wisely. The change of rhythm can quickly open a gap that others would have trouble closing. Or it could be an effort on your part to get up to the person or group that's ahead of you. When you respond to a surge, slowly reduce the margin of distance, close the gap, and get back in contact, wary that another surge may be imminent.

I'll never forget one of the first world-class 10K races that I saw in person on a stadium track. All the runners had impressive credentials. The favorite was a runner who had won all his races that year. One of the other great runners surged ahead. The favorite gradually worked his way back up to the leader, who surged again just as the favorite caught up. This must have happened four or five times until, finally, the favorite couldn't respond. The person who surged all those times won the race. It couldn't have been an easy race for either the winner or the favorite. To see this play out over those 25 laps was highly entertaining. The favorite did everything he could. He didn't sprint to reconnect with the leader, as that would have been a mistake. He would gradually close the gap to cover the move. On this day, the winner had one more move than the favorite.

## FINISH

A strong finish is essential. How much energy should you save? Or should the finishing speed be a strong mental attitude that you know is there no matter how badly you feel? If you save a lot, you may have

**Eric Albright**
**UD athlete 1990-1994**
**Mens Cross Country team photo**
**IC4A Championship meet**
**Waveny Park, Connecticut, Fall 1990**
**(photographer unknown)**

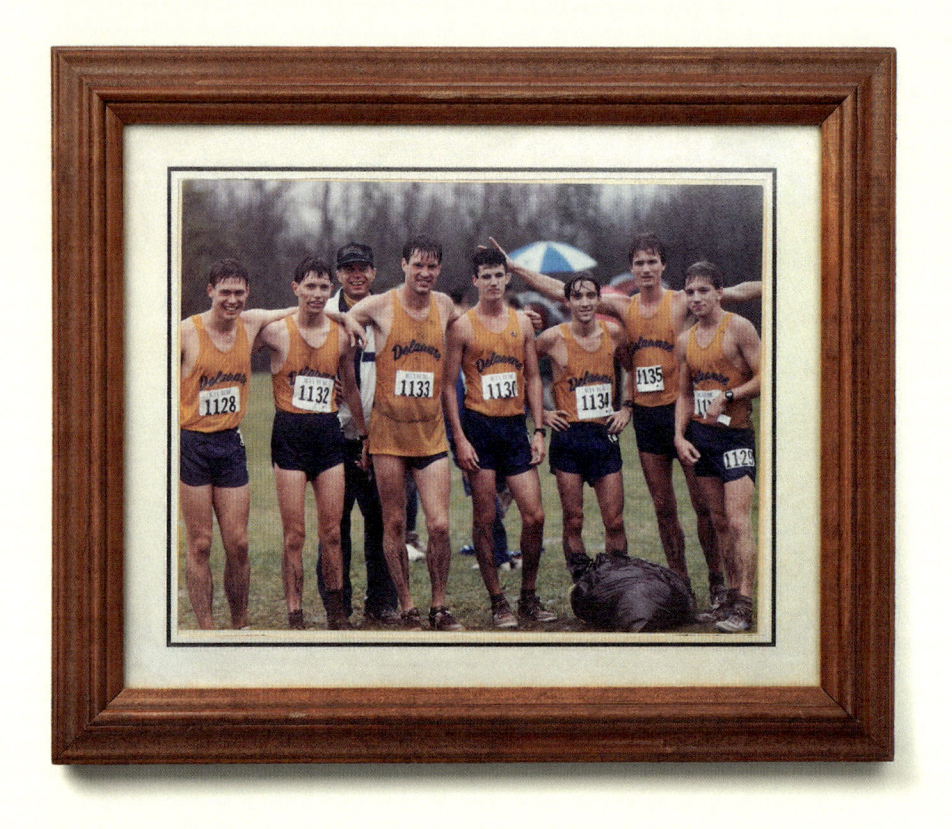

# Becoming a Team

**ERIC ALBRIGHT**

When I was deciding what college to attend and run for in 1989, my senior year of high school, I had a conversation with Coach Fischer. "We are looking to keep the best Delaware runners in-state and build something special here." Those words stuck with me, and I feel so fortunate that I chose to join Delaware cross country and track & field under the tutelage of Jim Fischer. For the next four years, I improved tremendously as a runner. More importantly, Fisch taught me lessons of life: humility, hard work, kindness, and compassion.

As a freshman, I didn't know what to expect from college running. I was intimidated but not overwhelmed. Fisch treated us all as equals, from fleet-footed Mark Tozer leading the pack to hard-working Michael Halbfish bringing up the rear. His belief in each of us gelled us as a team and allowed each of us to grow as a person and an athlete.

Fast forward a few months to our end-of-the-season XC championship. Fisch's dream of keeping some good runners in-state became a reality with our freshman class and was bolstered by some out-of-state talent from neighboring states. As the season progressed, that freshman unit remarkably became the core of the team. Eight of us would stick together for four years and, under Fisch's guidance, would take the team to a new competitive level.

There had been a LOT of rain leading up to the race; it was perfect cross country weather. I'll never forget coming around the first turn and seeing the course disappear into what looked like a lake. It was only ankle deep, but by the time we hit it, it had become sloppy and muddy. I don't think we had a great race that day, but we competed. Four of the seven runners that day were true freshmen. This picture captured that moment after the race. We knew we had something special. We knew we had a special coach!

already gone too slowly during the race and lost a lot of time. Spread the "hurt" out over the whole race. You should especially be in your "critical zone" frame of mind for the long drive to the finish. You might get challenged or passed near the finish, but you might also be racing against another "class" of runners much better than the ones you usually finish with. The training philosophy that I've outlined has been to complete every workout strongly. The mental image and the physical presence should be well established. Let that practice carry you over the finish line. It isn't a bad idea to save a little energy for the end of the race. However, sometimes it isn't about speeding up but holding your pace while everyone else is slowing down. I want you to be strong at the end, and most of all, I want you to know it, even when you are tired. This must be practiced over and over.

Make sure that you race through the finish line. The finish line is the finish line is the finish line. This needs to be practiced, practiced, and practiced every day. Easing your pace before you finish can cost you a victory, a place, a record, or a qualifying performance. Every race should be a strong effort for the whole distance, not a hard race for most of it, with a coast at the end. You want the pain to end as soon as possible. I get that. Just carry the strong pace for a few more seconds through the finish line. Always assume someone is on your heels, trying to pass you just before the finish line. How often have you seen someone in pain as they approach the finish line, seemingly going as fast as they can only to find another gear when challenged? Always go to that "other" gear.

Learning how to finish a race when you are tired, tight, or struggling is essential. You are almost sure to have a "bad patch." Some techniques for regaining control are dropping your arms and shoulders, calming your breathing, relaxing your upper body, shortening your stride length, quickening your rhythm, slowing down, and focusing on the people ahead of you. Hopefully, you will recover and be able to get going again. Avoid struggling to the finish without attempting to relieve the tightness and pain you are feeling. This is where mental toughness helps as long as you leave some of that mental space to help you finish faster. Float, grab some water or food (if available), and concentrate on your rhythm. Most of the time, you will work your way out of a bad patch and return to feeling more in control.

There can be only one winner. If everyone must be first, there will be many disappointed people. Remember, you aren't a failure if you fail to take first place. Figure out a plan, a way to be first, and give it your best shot. It is exceedingly rare that someone wins all the time. If you don't win, assess what happened and plan for a better result next time. If you are competitive and want to do well, your mental toughness may be your ticket. At some point during every tough race, the question will be asked: will I or won't I? Will you or won't you put up with the pain, and will you or won't you do what is necessary to be competitive? This is a quote that I remember from a long time ago, and I don't remember where I read it. "It is easy to find people who want to win. It is hard to find people who don't want to lose!"

After the race, keep moving with an easy run or walk. This will keep the heart and muscles working to bring oxygen and nutrients to the cells and take waste products away. Consume carbohydrates and some protein within the first 15 to 30 minutes post-race to help speed recovery. The rate of recovery is slower the longer you wait. Make sure you start drinking small amounts immediately and continue this at regular intervals. Start with water, especially if your digestive system is upset or overly sensitive. You might feel good right after the race, but your condition will deteriorate if you wait too long to rehydrate.

Change out of wet, sweaty clothes, including undergarments, as soon as possible. This is especially important in colder weather, where cold, wet, and wind can quickly drop your body temperature. Stretch, get a massage, roll out your muscles, eat small meals, hydrate, lie down and put your legs up against a wall, take an ice bath, and put on compression sleeves. These promote circulation and enhance recovery.

## RACING ON THE TRACK

Since there are so many turns in a track race, you should stay as close as possible to the inside of the lane without stepping on or inside the curb, rail, or lane line to run the shortest distance. There are caveats to this that will be explained later.

When in a race that starts in lanes where you will have to cut toward the inside of the track, stay in your designated lane or alley until you can legally cut to the inside. Then make sure you run a line directly to the inside lane of the next turn and don't cut sharply to the inside of the track immediately.

With championship meets, there is usually a fixed schedule of events, and each event will be run at a specific time. You know how much time you have until your event and can plan your warmup accordingly. However, many other non-championship meets have a rolling schedule; one event follows right after another with no specific times set. In this case, look at the number of heats with approximate time lapses. Determine a best-guess schedule and start your warmup accordingly. Warm up slowly with the thought that you could speed up or slow down the process if the meet were moving at a rate different than you had planned.

During a race, you must weigh the advantage of running the shortest distance versus protecting your position. Most people always want to run the shortest distance, but how much difference does it make? If you lose a close race, you may have a case. But if you get stuck in the inside lane and can't get out, that can be a serious problem.

Running the shortest distance on the inside may cause you to be boxed in or at least be in close quarters. You will run extra distance but be able to protect your position by running slightly behind the leader's outside shoulder. This can be a great place to be. You don't have to set the pace. You might get a little help with the wind. You won't get boxed in. You will force anyone behind you attempting to pass to go all the way around you. You can immediately tell if the leader speeds up. Watching the leader's outside shoulder will give you a consistent marker to focus on, keeping your head up rather than watching their feet. Now, you can easily make a move from that position to challenge for the lead.

The leader and anyone on the inside lane must be careful. If someone passes them to take the lead and another moves up beside the former leader, the former leader becomes boxed in and might have to wait and go out the back of the pack until everyone has passed and then pass runners on the outside. If you are the leader, "fill up your lane," so the trailing runners must decide if they want to go around you and add extra distance. Try to stay "free," even if you may run a little farther.

Be aware of your position and what is going on around you. If you are caught on the inside next to the rail with people all around, you must be patient and look for an opening. That's easier in a long race than in a short race or when you are near the finish line. If you are trapped, you can be more patient, for example, in a 1500m race than you can in an 800m race. Stay calm and try not to use nervous energy. Sometimes, the opening comes to the inside, but you do have to stay on the track. Another thing that you can do as you come off a turn is edge your way out and away from the curb. That might force the person outside you to move ahead or back if they don't want to run wide.

Passing on the curve is usually a bad idea when you want to make a pass. It takes a lot of effort, and you run quite a bit farther. However, waiting to initiate a pass until you are on the straightaway may not give you enough time to complete it before the next curve, especially on an indoor track. Anticipate and initiate a pass starting in the middle of the turn so that you are ready to go by the time you get to the straightaway.

Many times, there will be lapped runners in distance races. Let's say you are approaching a lapped runner and running on the inside next to the rail with someone running just to the outside of you. If you don't anticipate this, you might get caught behind the lapped runner while

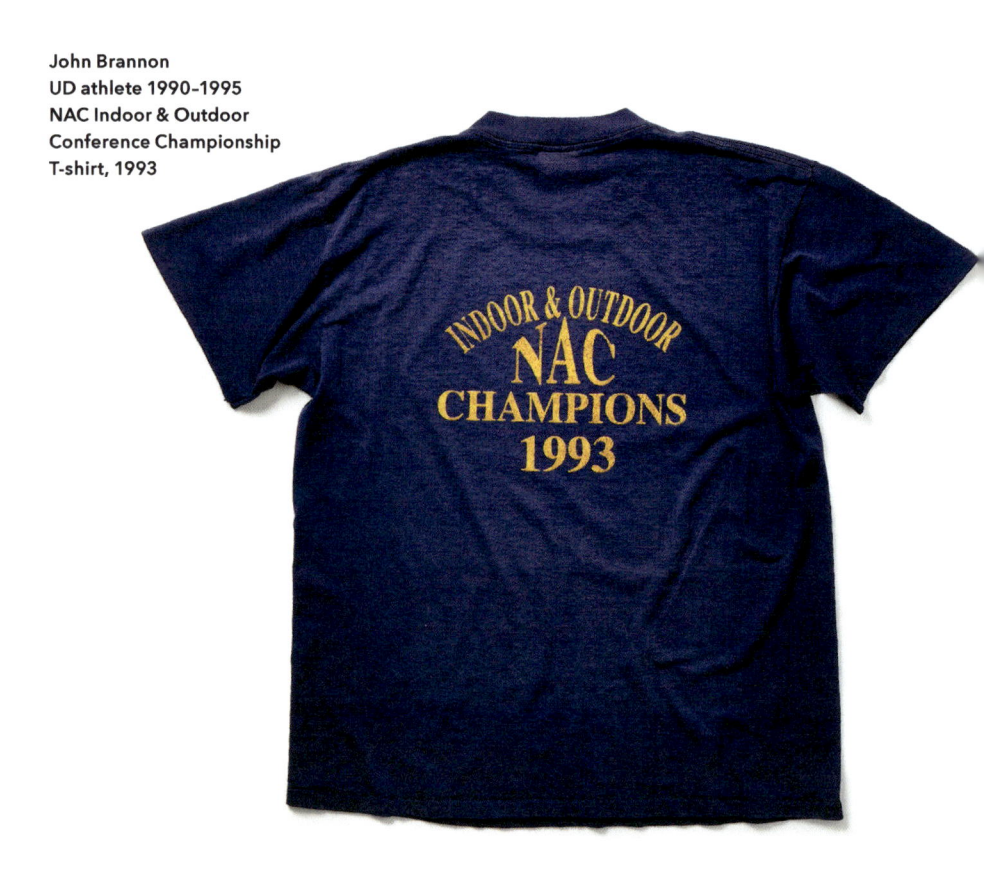

John Brannon
UD athlete 1990–1995
NAC Indoor & Outdoor
Conference Championship
T-shirt, 1993

## Champions and Friends

**JOHN BRANNON**

The 1993 Indoor & Outdoor Conference Champs T-shirt is worth keeping around for a long time, even if it looks like it's gone through a battle. I'm sure my former teammates can attest to that. Every time I look at the shirt, I think about some aspect of that 1993 season, but my mind usually comes back to the conference championship victory lap and being able to experience and enjoy that moment with all the coaches and teammates.

The everyday ups and downs of practicing and competing for the team were certainly enough to forever feel a strong sense of comradery and belonging, while the victory lap was the icing on the cake that made a particular moment and a group of people unforgettable.

178    RUN. TRAIN. RACE.

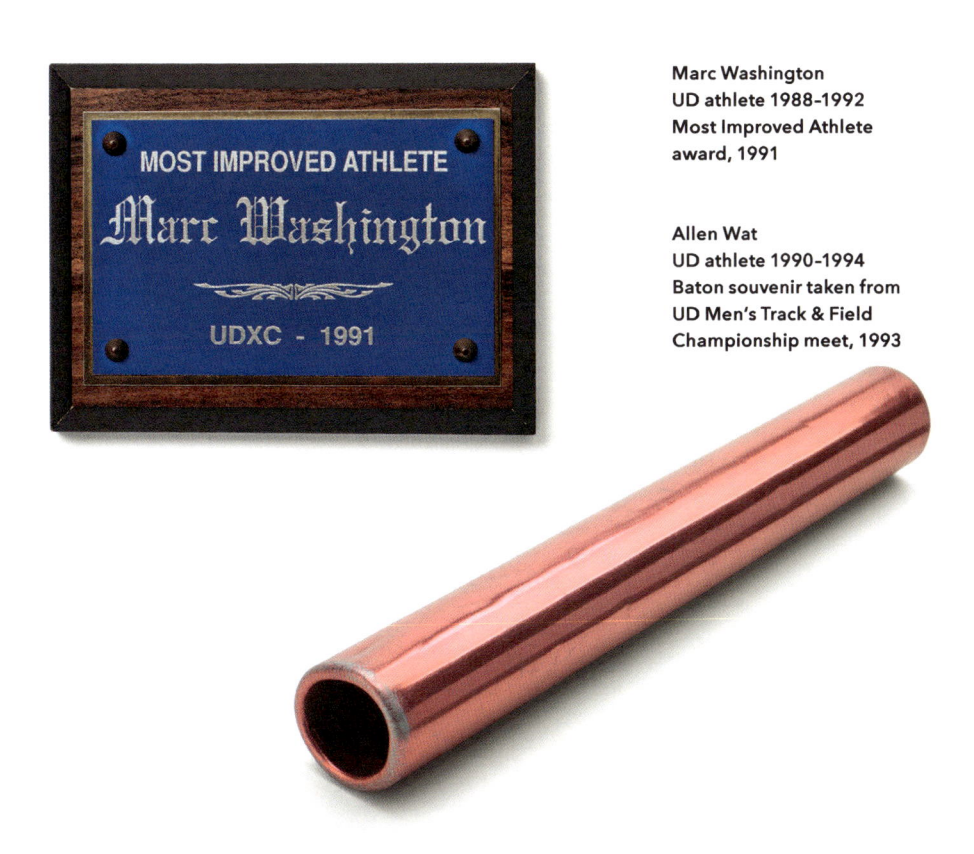

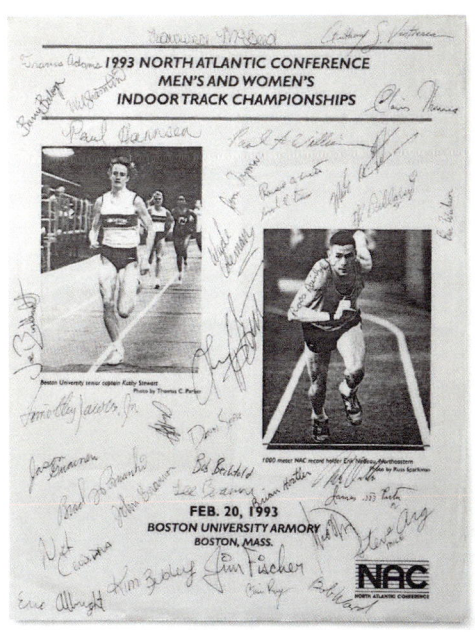

Marc Washington
UD athlete 1988-1992
Most Improved Athlete award, 1991

Allen Wat
UD athlete 1990-1994
Baton souvenir taken from UD Men's Track & Field Championship meet, 1993

Allen Wat
North Atlantic Men's and Women's Indoor Track Conference Championship program, 1993

RUN. TRAIN. **RACE.**

the person to your outside goes around them, leaving you behind. Either increase your pace to move ahead of the person running beside you to get around the lapped runner first or gradually move away from the curb, forcing the runner next to you farther outside. If you are the runner on the outside, you could anticipate passing the lapped runner first and speeding up. You could also slow down or hold your ground, forcing the runner on the inside to slow down.

There are times when you will be in a pack where you are the fastest person and other times when you will be the slowest, working hard to stay with the rest. This happens all the time with races split into sections. You may be just above or just below the cut-off line. Knowing the past performances of your competitors and how the event will be scored may change your strategy.

If you have multiple events on the same day, like at a track & field meet, eat and drink between events. Be aware of your time and ability to process the food. After an event, do a short warm-down jog, stretch, roll out, and massage your muscles, then jog a warmup, do striders, and mentally prepare yourself for the next one.

## RACING IN CROSS COUNTRY AND ROAD RACES

Road races are usually predictable, with a good surface, square corners, gradual hills, and nice start and finish areas. There are exceptions, but most courses have similar features. Cross country races are usually unpredictable, with uncertain surfaces, sharp turns, sudden narrowing, and steep hills. Both types of races require focus.

Cross country demands your attention. If you live close to the race site, practicing on the course will help you familiarize yourself with it to know what will come next and how to spend your energy. You may identify if there is a spot or two on the course where you may consider making a strong, confident move to take control of your race effort. Some racecourses have sections where you can recover/regroup. Other courses never give you a break. You want to know that ahead of time.

> If you don't become "one" with the course, it beats the crap out of you.

Gary Wilson
Former University of Minnesota
Women's Cross Country and
Track & Field Coach
Co-founder and executive director
of the Griak Invitational

If you have additional time, running the course backward can help you see the course and the hills from a different perspective.

During the warmup before a race, ensure you run the first and last half miles. It would be great to run the whole course. That isn't always possible. By running the first half mile, you can see if the course narrows, if there are issues with the surface, and where any early turns are located. The crowded start will make your vision difficult and limit your ability to move where you want. By running the last half mile, you will know where you are relative to the finish line and where you can start your final push. Too many times, I've seen people on the wrong side of a turn. They hit a muddy spot in a large group at the start or as the course suddenly narrows. I've also seen many misjudge how far they have left to reach the finish line.

A minor consideration, but something that might make a significant difference, is taking the shortest distance between two points. If a right turn is followed by a left turn or vice versa, in most cases, you will want to run diagonally, directly toward the next corner. It is called running the tangents. Don't stay in the middle of the trail or road or always on the same side of the course. The course is measured by the shortest path, the shortest distance possible. Any deviation from this principle means YOU ARE RUNNING LONGER!

There are a few more things you should know about turns. You will have many sharp turns. Pay attention if you are running in a group. We all want to run the shortest route. If you are in a group of runners, sometimes the person on the inside of the turn gets pinched and even stepped on. Setting yourself up on the outside of the group, even though you will run a farther distance, will allow you to anticipate a turn and either speed up or slow down to avoid a problem. This wise positioning will give you the space to make the turn free and clear and keep you moving without the stop-and-go and close traffic. If you are by yourself, there is a technique called "falling into the turn," where you shift your weight to the inside and slightly forward, which naturally causes an acceleration. Shaky footing and uneven balance would make this a bad idea. If there is a blind turn, you could use that to accelerate after the turn to widen the gap on someone behind you or accelerate into the turn to close the distance on someone ahead of you. Don't tell anyone about this. It will be our secret.

This is something that I mentioned before, and here it is again. When you are running up a hill, there are two ways to approach ascending it. You can maintain your effort, which will slow down your running speed, or you can maintain your running speed, increasing your effort. There are situations when you might want to do one and other times when you want to do the other. Practice them both. It will make a difference where the hill comes in the race, how long, how steep, how tired you are, and the location of your competition. Learn to accelerate into the hill ten to 20 meters before it starts. The more times you have practiced all of this, the better your instincts will be for the decision-making process. Most runners will want to take a breather once they reach the top. Running over the top or continuing to push once you have reached the top may open a gap that your competitors won't be able to close for the rest of the race. However, if you haven't practiced doing that and don't know how it will feel, it may be a wrong strategic decision. Sometimes, you must go hard and tolerate the pain anyway.

The crown or shape of the road can be troubling and bring on aches and pains. The repeated pounding can make for acute pain and discomfort. It can be debilitating. I've used the crown to my advantage a few times. If one of my legs started hurting, I would move to the center of the road or the other side where the slant was different to see if it would diminish or eliminate the pain. It didn't always work. It worked on enough occasions to make it worth trying.

When running long races, especially long road races, consider the tenets of the critical zone protocol. Try to get through the first two-thirds to three-fourths of the race, getting good position and using as little energy as possible. The last third of the race can feel bad if your energy is

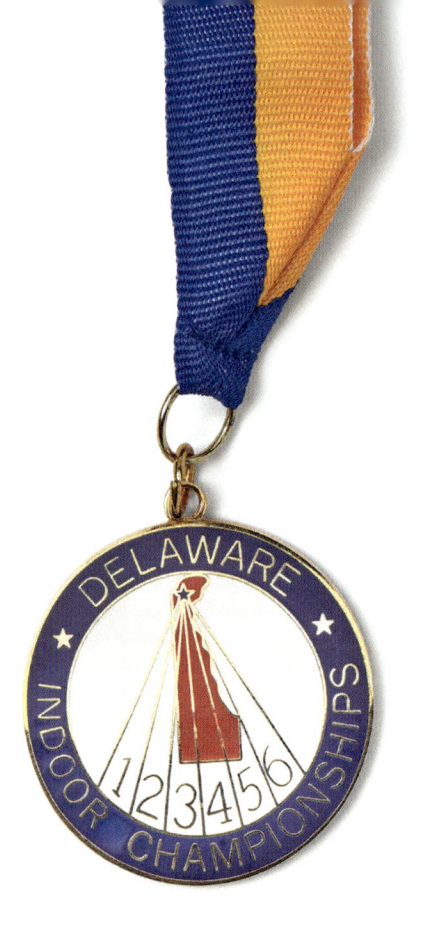

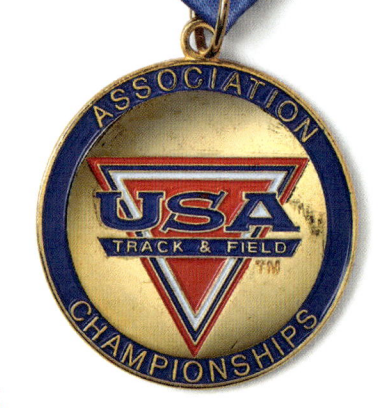

# Medals and Awards

**JIM FISCHER**

The dialog surrounding medals and awards is extensive, with opinions ranging from those who attribute significant value to them to others who argue that the value diminishes when everyone receives recognition. Both perspectives have valid points, and strongly favoring one side over the other is unnecessary.

An award is a commendation for high skill levels, commitment, strategy, and hard work, culminating in outstanding competitive results. In such cases, it is appropriate to congratulate and celebrate the individual for their exceptional performance.

Simultaneously, many of us harbor personal goals and aspirations. A participation award from an event can serve as a meaningful memento, commemorating a milestone,

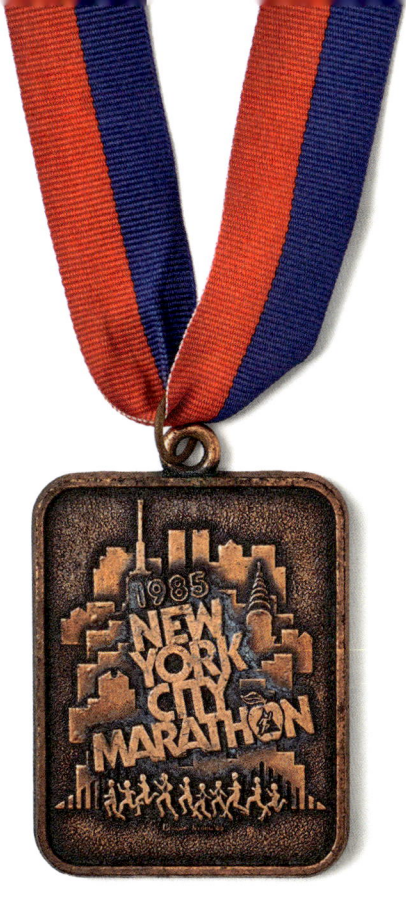

Jim Fischer
Four of the many medals collected over the course of my career

destination, or life event that holds significance for the individual. While I may have received recognition from events that held little personal value, for someone else, it could represent the pinnacle of their long journey. Reflecting on my own experiences, there are events I wish I had a tangible reminder of, as they held profound significance in my life, whereas for others, the same events might have been just another day.

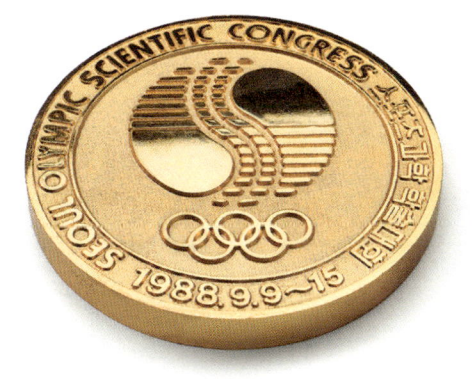

RUN. TRAIN. **RACE.**

drained. Plus, you will feel much better passing people rather than being passed. If you start to feel like you are struggling, don't be afraid to run with walking breaks so you can keep moving and get to the finish as soon as possible.

Make sure that you have practiced drinking from a cup while running. You need fluids. If it isn't a problem when you practice, great. I can't count the times when the fluids have gone up my nose, and I didn't swallow anything. I learned to squeeze the cup, forcing the fluids in, which helped. If you have trouble drinking while racing, you can walk a few steps just after the fluid stops. Pay attention to how you and your digestive system react to the fluids. You need energy at the end of the race. However, that is when the digestive system is usually most sensitive. There are times when sports drinks don't sit well. You could cut them with an additional cup of water. How many drinks, gels, chews, candy, or whatever can your stomach take? You have already had a long, hard day. During your training, devise a strategy for getting the energy you want and the fluids you need into your body.

## GETTING TO THE RACE

One of the best reasons to do some developmental races is to prepare for the race procedures and atmosphere. The paragraphs below will give you some things to consider to see what works for you and what doesn't.

Plan and pack before going to a race. Ensure you have tried on your racing outfit and shoes well before race day. Do a few workouts to break them in and see how they feel. Pack everything you might need. You want to avoid surprises on race day. I have an example of why this is important. This happened when we took a weight thrower to the national indoor track & field meet. It was the national meet, so we expected the throwing circle with normal conditions to throw from. We arrived and discovered the throwing surface was a polished cement floor. It was hard to walk on without slipping, let alone trying to throw a heavy weight from it. A shoe with a lot of grip is what was needed. It taught me a lesson. Take everything for every possibility with you. If you don't have it, you can't wear it. The surface you are running on may be one way during practice and completely different after a torrential downpour. Be prepared for whatever conditions that might occur. Take everything you have—clothes, food, drink—to the race site for every reasonable possibility you might need on race day.

If you must travel a long distance by air or in a car, walk around at least every two hours. Do everything you can to help the circulatory system and to loosen and stretch muscles. The air can be very dry on an airplane, so stay hydrated. When traveling over time zones, you can gradually change your light, eating, sleeping, and activity schedule to the new time zone before you go, keep your usual schedule once you get there, or travel to the site far enough in advance for your body to make the adjustments. Changes in heat, cold, humidity, or altitude will have dramatic effects. Acclimatization by early travel, two weeks, is the best case. For most of us, that isn't practical.

The following is the actual content of an itinerary for a cross country meet we were flying to. There was a banquet the night before, so I wrote the following note to the athletes along with their itinerary. "Please remember: uniform, shoes (training and racing), Friday workout clothes, Friday banquet clothes (nice), Saturday morning shakeout clothes (two to four miles easy at the hotel), Saturday warmup clothes, Saturday meet clothes, Saturday warm-down clothes, Saturday fly home clothes, a towel, pillow, cold weather gear, warm weather gear, rain gear, cap or hat, gloves, snacks, and anything else you might need. Take your shoes and racing uniform in your carry-on." One concern I didn't mention is that racing shoes with sharp spikes may not be allowed in a carry-on on the plane. Make sure that you plan for every possibility. Bring anything and everything you might need with you to the event.

On race day, do a short shakeout and eat three to four hours before race time, with younger kids eating a little closer to race time. That gives you enough time to process the food and go to the bathroom. Bagels,

# Get to the race rested and healthy.

bananas, cereal, peanut/almond butter, sports drinks, water, gel packs, and chews are typically good for most people. Know this ahead of time. Stay away from fats, fiber, and a lot of protein. A small amount of protein can be good, but a lot can be hard to digest. Limit dairy. Eggs, meats, fats, and fiber can cause problems, so avoid them. Some react badly to acidy or sugary drinks. Test these ahead of race day. It is odd to hear about people not eating on a marathon day, and it is particularly bad if the starting time is late. I've heard of athletes taking in little food before an afternoon or evening competition. That's putting them at a deficit.

On the other hand, if the pre-meet meal is too big, blood is diverted to the digestive system. Once running begins, if there is food in the digestive system, it is like a bag of food bouncing up and down. It isn't a good situation. Limit high fiber, fat, and protein as it could cause gastrointestinal distress.

Arrive at the race site well before the starting time. Try to be there at least an hour before, longer for a large race. Give yourself time to pick up your race number, go to the bathroom, and warm up. If it is a big race with long lines at the bathrooms, you might have to use the bathroom and get right back in line. Make sure to do enough of a warmup before the race and a good warm-down after. Use powder and blister gels on your feet and in your shoes, especially if you are running in a long race or on a rainy or hot and humid day. Blisters can't be a concern during the race. You should test this during practice sessions for long workouts in hot and humid conditions. Tie your shoes and run around in them to be sure they aren't too loose or too tight. If they feel good, double-knot them so they won't come undone. Remember that during a long race, your feet will swell.

In summary, be trained for the race distance, plan your diet for before, during, and after the race, make a schedule for race weekend including pre- and post-race, be confident in your preparation, be sure to cover all weather and running surface variables, be in control during your race, and enjoy yourself.

## RACE DAY

I'll give you my quick summary leading up to your race day. This is for THE race. This outline is the main setup for a road race with almost everything applicable to all races. And it starts long before race day.

- Do the whole training cycle. No shortcuts.
- Never do anything or wear anything for the first time on race day.
- Do developmental races to help you determine your strengths and weaknesses, strategies, race day procedures, rituals, and routines.
- Determine your sensitivity and timetable for eating pre-race.
- Practice drinking from a cup while you are running.
- Practice taking sports drinks, gels, chews, candy, or whatever you like during your longest and hardest workouts.
- Run your last long run three weeks before your goal race.
- Do your last hard workout eight to ten days before the race.
- Taper your training before the race to get the rest you need for race day.
- Try on your racing outfit and racing shoes two to three weeks before race day.
- Pack everything you need the day before and check it twice.
- Sleep well in the weeks leading up to race day. With tense nerves the night before a race, the best sleep night is two nights before.
- Study the course map and elevation chart ahead of time if it is provided.
- Learn what will be given out as refreshments before, during, and after the race to know how it affects you.
- Eat well, especially in the last few weeks before race day.
- Hydrate well. Drink one to two cups of water two hours before the race. You can have small amounts closer to race time.
- Monitor your fluid intake so you don't have to use the bathroom just before the start.
- Check your race number/chips three times before leaving for your destination.
- For extended travel to the race site, drink regularly, stand up, and stretch every hour or two.
- Eat a healthy meal the night before adding more carbohydrates and decreasing fats and fiber.

- Do a shakeout run three to four hours before the start of the race.
- After the shakeout, eat mainly easily digestible carbohydrates and take in fluids.
- Take a quick shower to feel fresh before wearing your racing uniform.
- Arrive at the race site at least an hour before the start time for a small and longer for a large race. Get your race packet as soon as you get to the site.
- Make sure you have extra clothes (that you could throw away) for cold weather, rain, or shade and extra fluids for hot weather.
- Leave your socializing until after your race. Greetings are fine.
- With long bathroom lines, there will be times you might have to go and get right back into the line. Bring toilet paper, just in case.
- Run a progressive warmup for short races, including the first and last 800m of the course.
- For long races, the early miles can be part of your warmup.
- Finish your warmup with strong, controlled striders.
- Take any nutrition that you want during the race with you.
- Position yourself in your assigned starting area.
- Make sure to double-knot your shoes.
- Don't go crazy when the gun goes off. Don't sprint to every open spot to run free and clear. Be patient until the crowd thins out and you have room to run.
- Have a Plan A, Plan B, Plan C, and Plan D. Run with intelligence and strong will!
- Pace yourself to pass people during your critical zone rather than being passed.
- If you are in a long race and start to feel like you are struggling, ease back, float, or take short walking breaks to keep moving to finish.
- After the race, keep moving with an easy run or walk.
- Stretch, get a massage, and eat a small meal of protein and carbohydrates soon after you finish.
- Change out of wet, sweaty clothes, including undergarments, as soon as possible.
- Glow in the aftermath!
- Thank the people who supported you.

## THE FOLLOWING IS A SIMPLE RACE DAY SCHEDULE I'VE USED WITH TEAMS

| | |
|---|---|
| 90 minutes | Be at the meet site |
| 60 minutes | 5-minute easy jog |
| 55 minutes | Drills and get water/sports drink |
| 45 minutes | 10-15-minute progressive warmup |
| 30 minutes | Stretch, get water/sports drink, use bathroom, change shoes (double knot), braid hair |
| 10 minutes | Go to the starting line, do striders, say a prayer, give a cheer, get ready |
| 0 minutes | Race Time! |
| After the race | Minimum 10-minute warm-down, eat recovery food, hydrate, change out of all wet and sweaty clothing |

After you have done all the training and everything else you could do, the main element is this: Get to the race rested and healthy! This gives you the best opportunity to have a great experience!

I wrote this book to have something for myself. I am summarizing how I coached and put down on paper the thoughts I had while working with runners of all ages for over 50 years. Indeed, some day-to-day things did not make it into the book. I wanted to print the things I felt were essential and give background information on why you do things and when. I enjoyed going back over 50+ years of notes, workouts, conversations with coaches, and interactions with the runners. It was hard to see an end point when I started, as everything seemed overwhelming.

I hope that everyone learns at least one thing from each of the three chapters. As Coach Gagliano told me years ago, I say to you now that I don't have any secrets. I have always enjoyed putting the puzzles together. My joy has been seeing success, whether improvements, championships, or reached goals of all kinds. The smiles of realization that the "impossible" has been achieved is a thrill that lasts a long time. I have been blessed to have been able to do something in my life that I have profoundly and thoroughly enjoyed. I hope that you will find the same joy in your own lives!

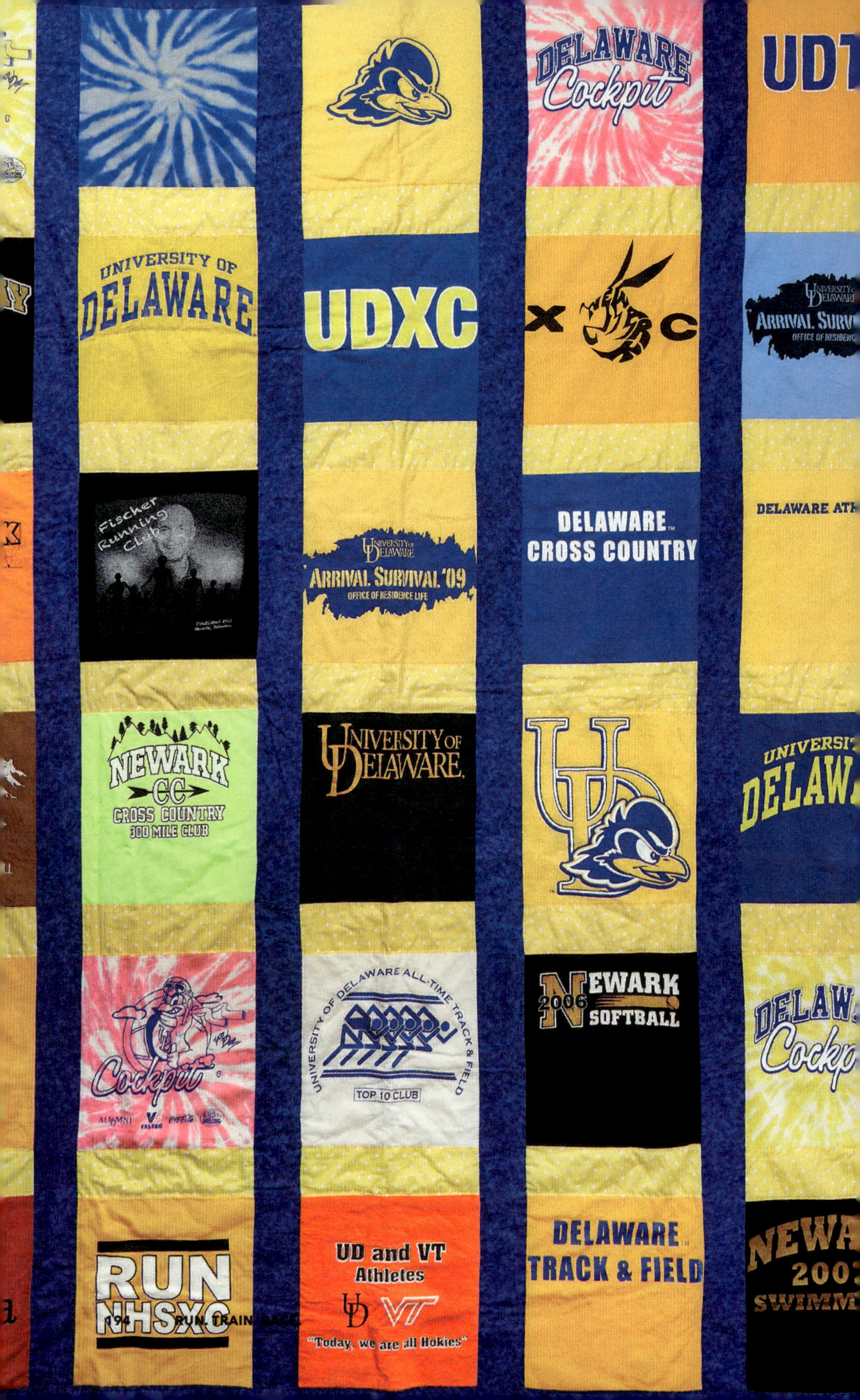

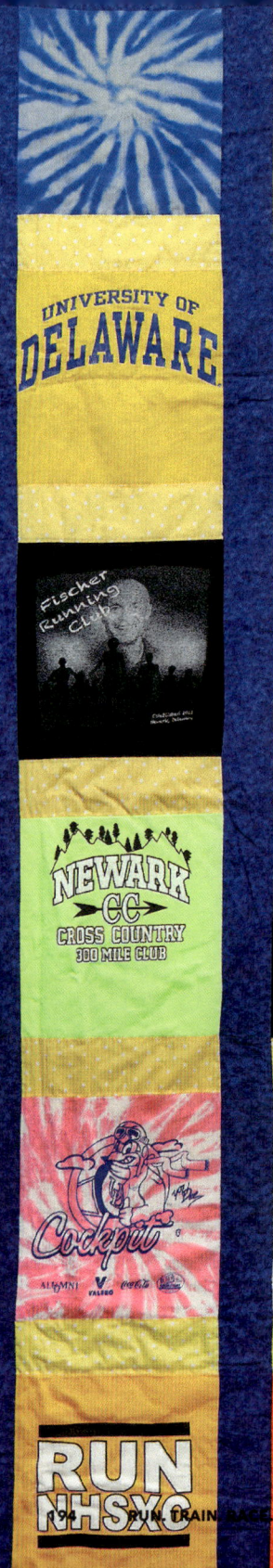

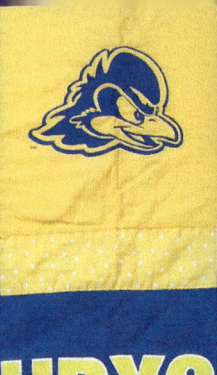

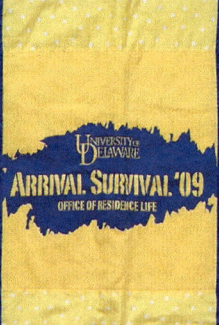

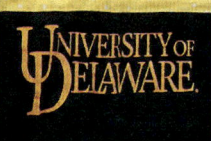

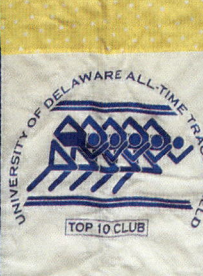

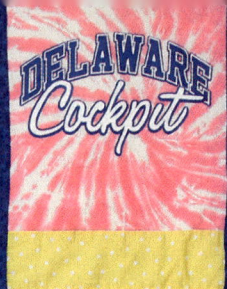

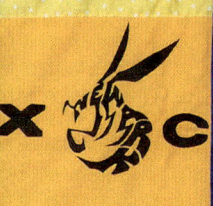

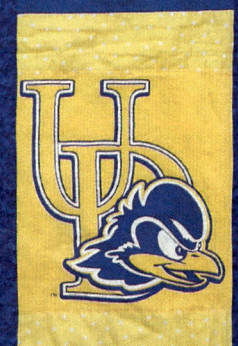

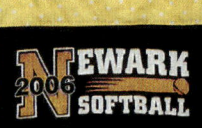

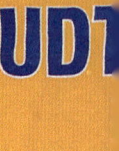

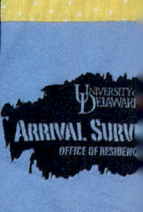

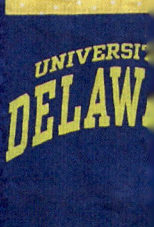

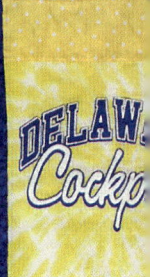

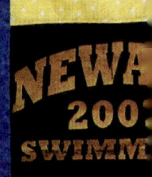

## WORKOUTS

2-5 x [2-4 x 400m @ 3K / 200m jog] / 5 min is read as two to five sets of two to four repetitions of 400m at 3K pace with a 200m jog interval between repetitions. Take five minutes between sets.

| | |
|---|---|
| **BL** | Blast—very hard but controlled, not struggling |
| **BU** | Build-Up |
| **CD** | Cut Down (each rep get faster) |
| **F-F-F** | Fast-Float-Fast |
| **Fartlek** | Speed Play (undefined lengths and paces; can be defined like intervals) |
| **Float** | Maintain Race Rhythm with Relaxed Upper Body |
| **FR** | Fast Relaxed |
| **Goal** | Goal Pace |
| **IO** | Ins and Outs—FR on Straights and Jog or Float Curves |
| **RP** | Race Pace |
| **m** | meters |
| **min** | minutes |
| **sec** | seconds |

8-10 x 150m BU / 50m walk

10 x 150m CD / walk back

200s until dusk—continuous 200m FR / 200m jog

4 x 400m @ 800m goal / 5 min

8 x 400m @ 1600m−5 sec / 3 min

4-6 x 400m CD starting at current 1600m / 5 min

5-8 x 400m @ goal 1600m / 1 min

2-Person 5-mile Relay—alternating 400m

2-5 x [5 x 400m @ 5K / 100m jog] / 5 min

2 x [3-5 x 500m @ goal 5K / 1 min] / 5 min

3-5 x 500m (300m FR-200m @ 90%) / 5 min

3-5 x 500m (300m FR-1 min-200m @ 90%) / 5 min

2 x [5-8 x 2 min FR / 1 min] / 5 min

2 x [4-6 x 600m F-F-F / 200m] / 5 min

600s Variety—600m straight, 600m BU, 600m F-F-F, 600m BL—200-400m recovery

4 x 600m Relay

**Karen (Mandrachia) Piacente**
UD athlete 2007-2011
UD Memories T-shirt quilt
2007-2011

2–4 x 800m of 50s

2 x [3–6 x 800m—1st set @ 5K / 200m; 2nd set CD / 400m] / 5 min

3–5 x 800m (500m FR-1 min-300m @ 800m) / 5 min

3–5 x 800m (500m FR-300m @ 90%) / 5 min

3–5 x 800m (4 x 200m @ goal 800m / 1 min) / 5 min

3–5 x 4 min CD / 5 min

2 x [2–5 x 1000m @ 5K / 200m–400m] / 5 min

3–5 x 1000m CD / 5 min

3–5 x 1000m [200m @ 1600m-100m jog-400m @ 3K-100m jog-200m @ 800m] / 5 min

3–5 x 1000m (500m @ 1600m-200m jog-300m @ 800m) / 5 min

2–6 x 1200m @ 5K / 400m + 2–5 x 400m @ 1600m

3–5 x 1200m (800m @ 5K-400m @ 3K) / 5 min

2–4 x 1200m (4 x 300m @ 1600m / 1 min) / 5 min

2 x [2–4 x 1200m @ 5K / 400m] / 5 min

3 x 1500m (300m @ 1600m-100m jog-300m @ 1600m-100m jog-300m @ 1600m-100m jog-300m @ 1600m) / 5 min

3 x 1500m (500m @ 1600m-1 min-500m @ 1600m-1 min-500m @ 1600m) / 5 min

3–6 x 1600m @ 10K / 400m

1600m + 800m + 800m—all hard with full recovery

2–4 x 2000m (1000m @ 10K-1000m @ 5K) / 5 min

70-90s, 75-95s, 80-100s, etc.—sets or continuous—(alternating 400ms—1st @ sub 5K, 2nd @ 1st 400m time plus 20 seconds)

1600m @ 10K-1600m tempo-1200m @ 5K-1600m tempo-800m @ 3K-1600m tempo-400m @ 1600m

800m @ 5K-1600m tempo-800m @ 5K-1600m tempo-800m @ 5K-1600m tempo-800m @ 5K

Undefined Fartlek—let terrain, landmarks, and fatigue level dictate the intensity and recovery

30:30 Fartlek—5:00 @ 5K-6:00 tempo-3:45 @ sub 5K-6:00 tempo-2:30 @ 3K-6:00 tempo-1:15 @ 1600m

Continuously rotating single file—last person to the front

Ins and Outs—run the straights, jog the curves—continuous for total time

50s—alternating 50m with fast, then float

Hills—short and steep for speed and power, long and gradual for strength endurance

10–15 sec Sprint Hills

Progression Runs—gradually increasing the pace of a distance run

Tempo Runs—slightly faster than half marathon pace

Cruise Intervals—tempo paced or slightly faster, controlled, spaced with short recovery

Time Trials—individual events and relays

1200m @ 5K-2-mile tempo-1200m @ 5K-2-mile tempo-1200m @ 5K

200m + 400m + 600m + 800m + 600m + 400m + 200m with 200m-400m recovery—faster down

1–4 x [4 x (Jog 60 sec-Stride 45 sec-Controlled Quick 30 sec-Sprint 15 sec)] / 5 min

1 min + 2 min + 3 min + 4 min + 5 min + 6 min + 5 min + 4 min-3 min + 2 min + 1 min/equal time

400m + 800m + 1200m + 1600m + 2000m + 1600m + 1200m + 800m + 400m with 200m-400m recovery with 800m & 1200m @ 5K, 1600m & 2000m @ 10K—faster down

800m + 1200m + 1200m + 800m + 1200m + 1200m + 800m with 800m @ 3K–5K, 1200m @ 5K–5K+, 400m jog recovery

1600m & 1400m @ 10K / 400m + 1200m & 1000m @ 5K / 400m + 800m & 600m @ sub 5K / 400m + 400m & 200m @ 1600m / 200m

1 x 1600m @ 10K + 1–2 x 1200m @ 5K + 1–3 x 800m @ goal 5K + 1–4 x 400m @ 1600m-3K with 400m recovery for all

3–5 x 2800m (1200m @ 5K / 400m jog / 400m @ 1600m / 400m jog / 400m @ 1600m) / 5 min

600m + 800m + 1200m + 400m + 400m + 200m + 200m @ goal 1600m with 5 min recovery

400m + 600m + 800m + 300m + 300m + 200m + 200m @ goal 1600m with 5 min recovery

300m + 400m + 600m + 200m + 200m + 100m + 100m @ goal 800m with 5 min recovery

1-2 x [8 x 200m @ 1600m / 1 min] / 5 min

2–4 x 1200m (4 x 300m @ 1600m / 1 min) / 5 min

3 x 1500m (300m @ 1600m-100m jog-300m @ 1600m-100m jog-300m @ 1600m-100m jog-300m @ 1600m) / 5 min

3 x 1500m (500m @ 1600m-1 min-500m @ 1600m-1 min-500m @ 1600m) / 5 min

2–4 x 2000m (1200m @ 5K / 400m jog / 400m @ goal 1600m) / 5 min

2–4 x 2000m (1000m @ 10K-1000m @ 5K) / 5 min

2000m or 3000m @ 10K + 5 min + 2 x 1000m CD / 5 min + 5 min + 2–4 x 400m @ 1600m / 400m

Colin McMillan
Race tag
Rock'n'Roll Half Marathon
Washington, DC
2018

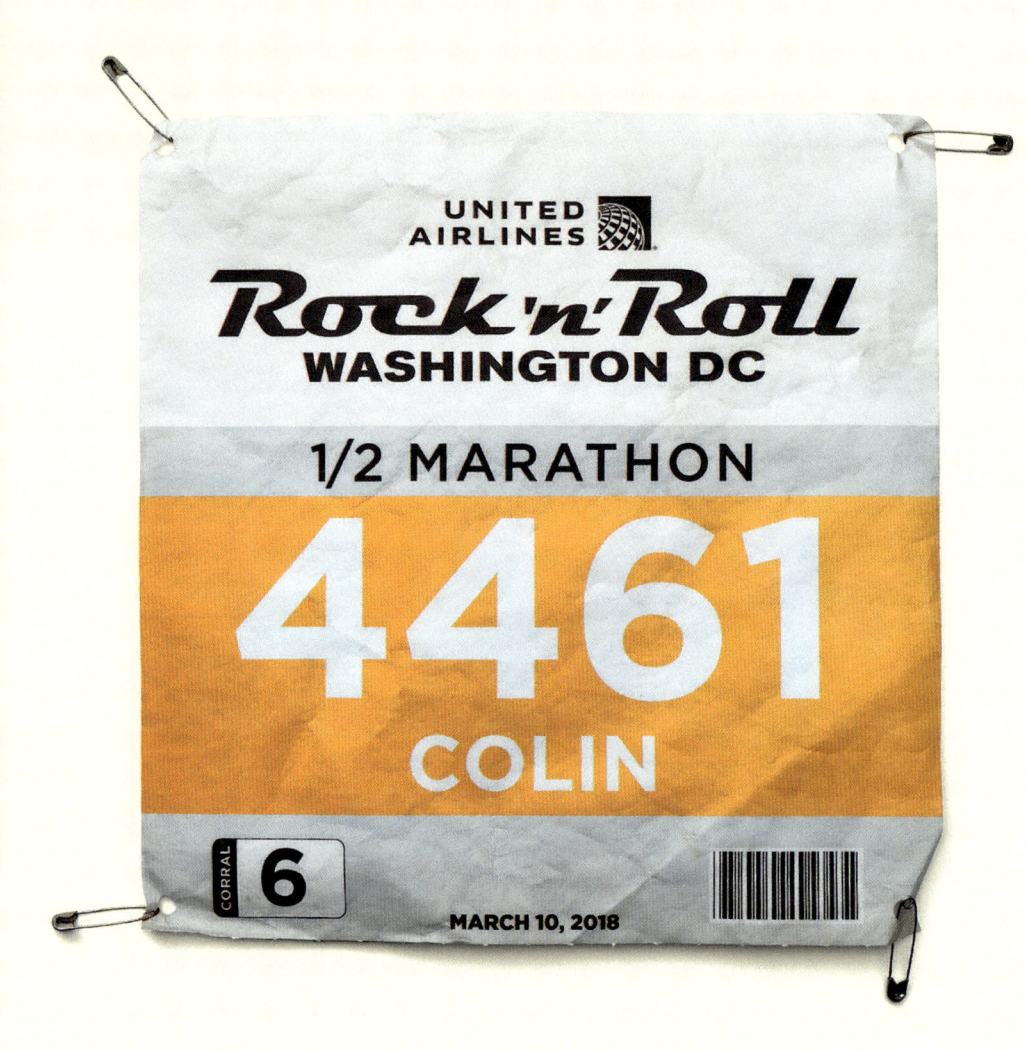

# Congratulations, Coach!

**LAURA MCMILLAN**

I never considered myself a "real" runner. As an athlete, my focus was on the field, not the track. But that changed when I read an early draft of this book. Jim's writing and his coaching captivated me, stirring curiosity and unearthing a potential I hadn't recognized.

Within a few months, I had taken everything to heart, introducing new workouts and embracing challenges, ultimately leading to my first half marathon. Before I knew it, I was completely hooked.

In 2022, I embarked on my most significant challenge yet: training for The Marine Corps marathon. Race day brought on a few tough lessons, typical for many first-time marathoners, and when I crossed the finish line, there were tears in my eyes. I had missed my goal by ten minutes. I had failed.

Frustrated and disappointed, I limped through the finishers' village until I finally spotted my parents. Among the crowd, it was Jim's smile that struck me. "That was amazing! You are amazing."

Once again, Jim changed my perception of myself. His positivity, pride, and encouragement provided exactly what I needed in that moment—the support of a coach who saw beyond numbers and results at the finish line. He recognized the months of unwavering dedication, hard work, and discipline that brought me to the start line, too.

I share this story because every runner under Jim's guidance has experienced this moment. He fosters a coaching environment rooted in inclusivity and respect, valuing and supporting every runner. Whether a novice (like me) or a seasoned athlete, Jim proudly celebrates the journey to the start line and everything it takes to cross the finish line.

It's only fitting that now, we get to celebrate you. Congratulations, Coach!

Our ambitions take us places—good and bad. When we are ambitious about friendship, we are on the right track, we are moving with the right rhythm, and we end up in the right place.

Rev. Dr. Nate Phillips

## ACKNOWLEDGMENTS

Since I started this project, I have had numerous chances to reflect on my career. Many people have guided me through all my years of coaching. Mentors who have directly impacted my knowledge include Frank Gagliano, Roy Griak, Harry Groves, Art Gulden, Bill Guy, Rick Kleyman, Bill Thomson, and Charles Torpey. I have learned much through lectures from and conversations with Beth Alford-Sullivan, Scott Christensen, Vin Lananna, Don Larson, Rod Olson, Steve Plasencia, Mike Poehlein, Al Schmidt, Boo Schexnayder, Paul Schmaedeke, Gordon Thomson, Robert Vaughan, Greg Watson, and Gary Wilson. Thanks for the years of support I received from Dr. Kathryn Carroll. I gained broad knowledge and insight from working side by side with Melanie Aube, Patrick Castagno, Joe Compagni, Nadine Marks Dempsey, Terri Dendy, Mike DiGennaro, Kevin Fauntleroy, Dick Fischer, Tom Fischer, Michelle Flanagan, John Flickinger, Marnie Giunta, Brittany Keller, Kevin Kelly, Wendy McFarlane-Smith, Sue McGrath-Powell, Bob O'Hara, Cindy Seikkula Peterson, Larry Pratt, Andrew Rudawsky, Vicki Huber-Rudawsky, Pete Schuder, Rick Schuder, and Stephanie Scalessa Whitby. I must also mention the athletes who taught me daily about pushing limits and making adaptations in training.

Many people helped me with this book. Brittany Keller and Linda Reisor edited it, Christine Fischer designed it, and Carlos Alejandro was the photographer. I want to thank friends who made valuable suggestions and contributed artifacts, stories, and quotes including Travis Adams, Eric Albright, Leah-Kate Atkinson, Melanie Aube, Dr. Elisa M. Benzoni, John Brannon, Jim Bray, Dr. Kathryn Carroll, Patrick Castagno. Joe Compagni, Jonathan Cooney, Gina Crist, Janet and Ed Davenport. Nadine Marks Dempsey, Mike and Dani DiGennaro, Dr. William Farquhar, Dick Fischer, Tom Fischer, Marnie Giunta, Art Gulden, Sarah Heins, Andre Hoeschel, Brittany and David Keller, Bill and Melissa Lafferty, Laini McGonigle, Laura and Colin McMillan, Rev. Dr. Nate Phillips, Karen (Mandrachia) Piacente, Steve Plasencia. Anna Pryor, Ron Reisor, Noel Relyea, Andrew and Vicki Huber-Rudawsky, Katarina Smiljanec, Liz Swierzbinski, Marc Washington, Allen Wat, Emily (Gispert) and Andy Weaver, Gary Wilson, and Bobby Zeidler. Words cannot express my appreciation for all your time and effort.

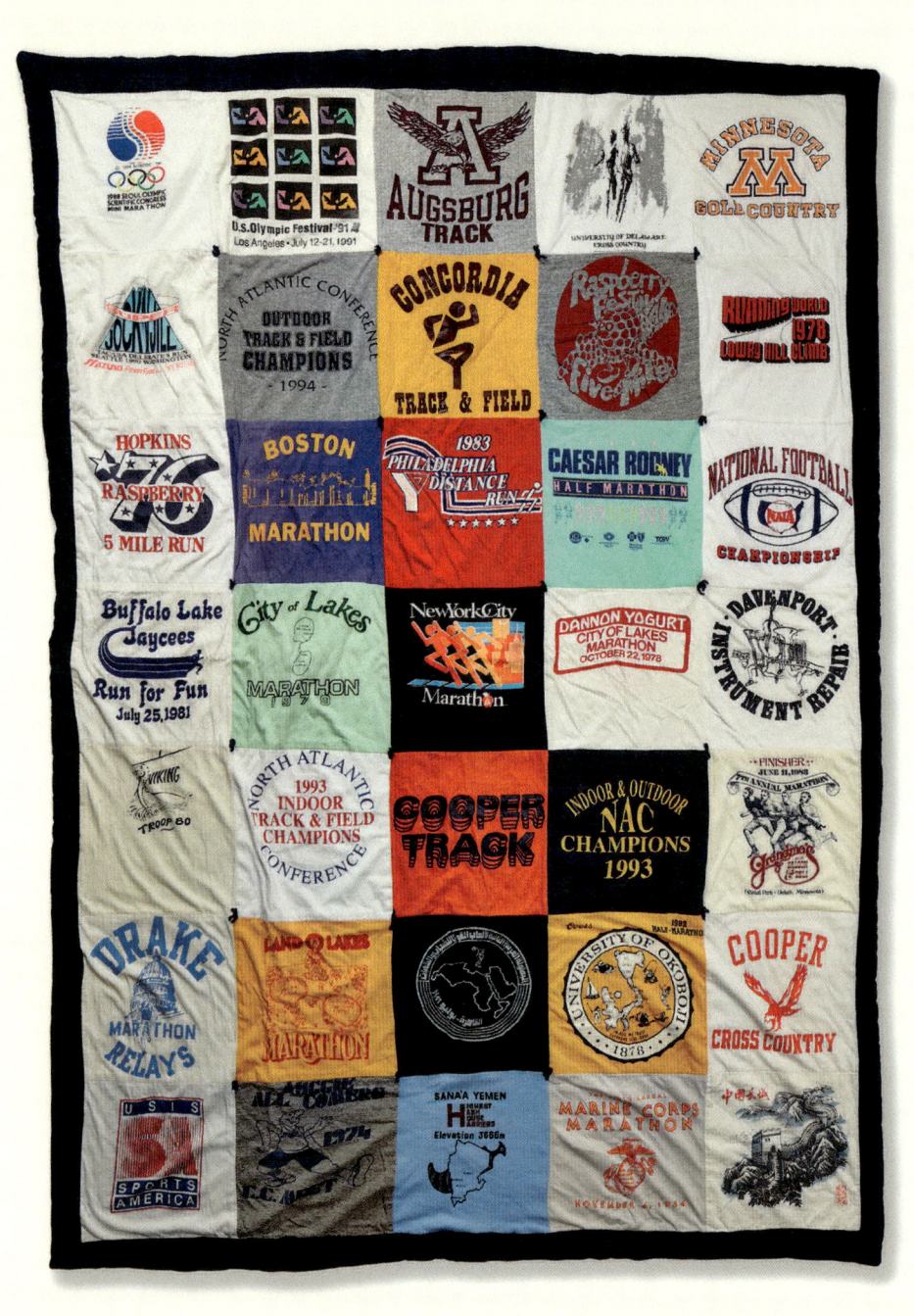

Jim Fischer
T-shirt quilt gift from
Dr. Kathryn Carroll
1996

202   RUN. TRAIN. RACE.

## ABOUT THE AUTHOR

Coach Fischer grew up in Buffalo Lake, Minnesota. He received a B.A. from Augsburg University and his M.Ed. from the University of Minnesota. He began teaching and coaching in Robbinsdale School District, a suburb of Minneapolis. He taught health and physical education while coaching cross country, track & field, cross country skiing, and basketball for over ten years. He assisted for one season at the University of Minnesota during that time. He then spent two years at Concordia College in Moorhead, Minnesota, as track & field coach and assistant football coach. In 1982, he joined the University of Delaware, where he spent 30 years as an Assistant Professor and cross country and track & field coach—45 of his teams placed in the top three at conference championships. After retiring from the University of Delaware, he coached at Delaware Technical and Community College, Sanford School and Ursuline Academy in Delaware. Under his leadership, Ursuline Academy won three consecutive State Championships team titles. For 40 years, he held weekly public training sessions for runners of all abilities. He ran 20 marathons and numerous other races. He served on the NCAA Men's Cross Country Coaches Association's Executive Board for 16 years, including two years as the president. He presented a paper on the "Biomechanical Profile of Elite Women Marathoners" in Seoul at the Seoul Olympic Scientific Congress, 1988. He is a Level III certified coach in endurance and has taught Level I and Level II certification classes in California, Louisiana, Maine, Maryland, Missouri, New York, Pennsylvania, and Washington. He has spoken at clinics in Delaware, Minnesota, New York, and Pennsylvania. He presented coaching and training clinics in China, Egypt, Honduras, and Yemen. He was an assistant coach for the "East Team" at the 1991 U.S. Olympic Sports Festival in Los Angeles. He co-founded the Delaware Track & Field Hall of Fame. He has worked with nonprofits, including the Leukemia & Lymphoma Society and Special Olympics, as well as running clubs and athletic organizations. He has been inducted into the Hall of Fame by six organizations and was named Delaware's Coach of the Year in 2020.

## BIBLIOGRAPHY AND RESOURCES

Dick, Frank W., 1991, *Training Theory*, British Amateur Athletic Board

Bompa, T. O., 1994, *Theory and Methodology of Training*, 3rd edition, Kendall/Hunt

Daniels, Jack, 1998, *Daniels' Running Formula*, Human Kinetics

Olson, Rod, 2011, *The Legacy Builder*, Denali Press

Sheehan, George, 1976, "6 Steps Toward Painless Running," *Runner's World*. December

Gary Wilson, former University of Minnesota Women's Cross Country and Track & Field Coach, Co-Founder and Executive Director of the Griak Invitational, speaking with USTFCCCA Communications Manager Tyler Mayforth on the difficulty of the Griak Invitational cross country course

Consultations with Andrew Rudawsky on injuries and rehabilitation

Numerous lectures, discussions, panels, books, athletes, coaches